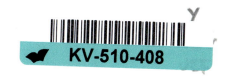
# Cancer: from cure to care

*Palliative care dilemmas in general practice*

POP

*David Jeffrey*

Published by Hochland & Hochland Ltd,
The University Precinct, Oxford Road, Manchester M13 9QA.

ISBN 1 898507 83 X

A catalogue record for this book is available from the British Library.

Printed in Scotland by Bell & Bain Ltd.

*Cancer: from cure to care*

# CONTENTS

*This book is dedicated to Pru.*

Acknowledgements

I thank the participating general practitioners for their honesty,
time and wisdom, and my wife Pru for her encouragement.

I am grateful to the following for financial support:
BMA Charles Hastings Award, the Royal College of General
Practitioners, The BUPA Foundation Communication Award
and the Department of Health for locum funding
under the extended leave programme.

# INTRODUCTION

*Vex not his ghost: O, let him pass! He hates him,*
*That would upon the rack of this tough world*
*Stretch him out longer.*

**William Shakespeare**

A patient may perceive a diagnosis of cancer as a sentence of death. Once cancer is diagnosed the patient's world becomes unpredictable. It is not only the prospect of a premature death, but the possibility of an undignified, painful process of dying, which may be frightening for the patient.

Cancer care can be divided into phases which reflect the aims of treatment: curative, palliative and terminal.[1]

## Curative care

Earlier diagnosis of cancer and advancing medical technology have generated high expectations amongst patients of medicine's power to cure. Such expectations may be fuelled by media reports of 'breakthroughs' in cancer treatment, by medical optimism, or by a cultural fear of death.

At the time of Hippocrates, holistic health and cure was thought to result from spiritual wellbeing. The purpose of medicine was not to identify localised lesions but to explain illness in terms of the total mental and physical disposition of the patient. The linking of the term 'cure' to medical treatment developed in the seventeenth century with the advent of the Cartesian revolution. This dualistic philosophy separated the workings of the mind and body. 'Cure' then became associated with the removal of physical disease, ignoring the subjective aspects of illness.[2]

The scientific advances of the twentieth century have encouraged oncologists, radiotherapists and cancer surgeons to adopt a biological view of cancer. There is now a risk of cancer being perceived as an organ dysfunction rather than an illness which affects the whole person.

Moreover, doctors are now involved in many areas of people's lives. Experiences such as ageing, dying and bereavement are now matters for medical concern and control.[3] Illich, a critic of this trend, argues that modern medicine's power to harm extends beyond the side effects of aggressive treatments to include the dependence of people upon doctors to solve all their problems.[4] He maintains that one consequence of this medicalisation is that death has come to be seen less as an inevitable part of life, and more as a failure of treatment.[4]

The technology which has given doctors the potential to cure certain cancers has also allowed them to prolong the process of dying. Thus a tension exists between the availability of life-prolonging treatments with significant side effects and a desire to resist the use of such therapies where the quality of life of the patient cannot be maintained. If patients from cancer are to receive appropriate care there is a need to explore the process and outcomes of medical decision-making.

## Palliative care

In contrast to the biological view of cancer treatment, in the palliative phase, emphasis is placed as much on the subjective feelings of the patient and the impact of the illness on the social, emotional and spiritual aspects of his life, as on the physical disease.

Palliative care is defined as the active total care of patients whose disease is not responsive to curative treatment. Control of pain, of other symptoms and of psychological, social and spiritual problems is paramount. The goal of palliative care is achievement of the best quality of life for patients and their families. Many aspects of palliative care are also applicable earlier in the course of the illness in conjunction with anticancer treatment. Palliative care neither hastens nor postpones death; it provides relief from pain and other distressing symptoms, integrates the psychological and spiritual aspects of care, and offers a support system to help the family cope during the patient's illness and in bereavement.[5]

In the palliative phase there is a shift in emphasis from quantity of life to quality of life.[6] This shift has a important consequence: a requirement to listen to the patient's views. The recognition of the existence of a natural dying process is central to the ethics and practice of palliative care.

Much of the philosophy and knowledge of palliative care was developed within the hospice movement. The establishment of hospice care represents a compromise between the over-enthusiastic application of technology to prolong life and the realisation that many dying people do not wish to endure the personal indignities these technologies may involve.[7]

## Terminal care

Terminal care refers to the last days of life. In this phase, the aim of care is to enable the patient to die with dignity. Harmful or distressing side effects of treatment are not acceptable.[1]

The first step towards the improvement of the care of patients with advanced cancer in the community is to define the problems encountered in providing palliative care.

I begin with a description of a qualitative study to discover what general practitioners felt were the main difficulties and uncertainties which arose in providing palliative care in the community.

Having gained an understanding of these difficulties and uncertainties, each is analysed with the aim of suggesting how these problems may be addressed.

Finally I explore medical decision-making and suggest some new ways of handling the uncertainties which arise in palliative care.

I hope that this book will stimulate debate between healthcare professionals and with patients and their families as to what constitutes the most appropriate care. Although primarily for healthcare professionals, the book may be of interest to anyone who wishes to increase their understanding of the dilemmas encountered in the care of patients with advanced cancer. With greater understanding we can work together to derive more appropriate ways of providing palliative care.

*David Jeffrey*

# LISTENING TO THE
# GENERAL PRACTITIONER'S TALE

*Where is the understanding we have lost in knowledge?*
*Where is the knowledge we have lost in information?*

T S Eliot

Traditionally, general practitioners have a wealth of anecdotal data on patients and their illnesses. This book seeks to answer questions which arise partly because patients, doctors, nurses and relatives have different beliefs, values and feelings about what constitutes the best way to treat a patient with advanced cancer. A qualitative approach is used to research the doctors' experiences, attitudes and uncertainties in caring for patients with advanced cancer at home.

Much of the everyday work of general practitioners involves decisions that are qualitative rather than quantitative.[8] Qualitative research can explore aspects of complex behaviour, attitudes, and interactions which quantitative methods cannot.[9,10,11]

In qualitative research the concepts of reliability and validity which are integral to quantitative research may be replaced by a notion of 'trustworthiness'. Thus the validity of observational accounts relies on the truthful and systematic presentation of the research. In many ways it is honesty which separates this observational account from a novel.[12]

Triangulation is one method of ensuring validity of qualitative data. A wide range of different sources of data are compared. In this study common themes emerged from the GPs reflecting on their care of different patients. The findings were returned to the participants to see if they regarded them as a reasonable account of their experiences. The study also includes 'negative' data or 'deviant cases' where the researcher's explanatory scheme is contraindicated.[13] The conclusions from the study are compared to experience cited in the literature.

Focus group sessions with other healthcare professionals also raised concerns which were congruent with those of the study general practitioners.

However, there are limitations to qualitative research. As Reinharz said, 'I will never know the experience of others, but I can know my own, and I can approximate theirs by entering their world. This approximation marks the tragic, perpetually inadequate aspect of social research.'[14]

Traditionally doctors have used anecdotes and case discussions as a valuable source of learning.[15] The challenge for the researcher is to translate this raw qualitative experience into objective data.

The critical incident technique described by Flanagan is one way of meeting this challenge.[16] This technique focuses the general practitioner on the specific problem which is being studied and thus reduces variability, subjectivity and unreliability.[15] In-depth interviews are a way of gaining access to the private, often contradictory beliefs people hold.[9] Case studies are valuable where broad, complex questions have to be addressed in complex circumstances.[8]

Two urban general practices which were involved in general practice vocational training were invited to participate. Practice 1 involved four male partners and one female partner, practice 2 comprised three male partners and three female partners.

In both practices, all patients over the age of 18 who died with a diagnosis of cancer during a complete year were included in the study. Summarised case histories of each patient were prepared by the researcher and given to their doctors who then chose a case (or cases) which they wished to discuss. Seventeen cases were selected for detailed discussion.

The next stage was a semi-structured interview with the researcher. The GPs were asked to reflect on issues of uncertainty or difficulty with particular reference to their cases. The case histories acted as a trigger to explore more general concerns. The interviews were taped and then transcribed verbatim by an experienced medical secretary and analysed by the researcher.

A critical incident was anything that the doctor felt was either an example of good practice or one which may have given rise to concern about the care the patient received, the quality of the patient's life and death and the quality of life of the surviving relatives or carers. The critical incidents formed natural clusters or categories.

A content analysis involves a process of developing categories from the transcripts. The transcripts were read and categories emerged which were common to many of the GPs stories. Using exact quotations to justify assignments of incidents to categories ensured that classification was based on the actual data and not on subjective judgements made on the basis of the researcher's views.

## Categories

The categories of problems which emerged included:

- Defining when palliative care begins
- Stopping active cancer treatments
- Communication with patients
    Breaking bad news
    Estimating prognosis
    Lack of time
    Maximising choice
    Talking about dying
    How to introduce specialist palliative care
- Communicating with relatives
- Communicating with hospital staff

- Symptom control problems
- Providing continuity of care
- A prolonged dying
- Promoting effective teamwork
- Sources of stress

There is a problem with presenting qualitative analyses because of the sheer volume of data. This study presents numerous sequences from the original data followed by a detailed commentary.[13]

At the time of the data collection I was a general practitioner from another town. I have subsequently become a specialist in palliative medicine.

# CHAPTER TWO

# THE BOUNDARIES OF
# PALLIATIVE CARE

*Perhaps they should have sat down and said look there really is no point in
doing this, that and the other, we really are treating symptoms. But she
always faced you with a joyous expression: 'OK, what can you do now?'*

General Practitioner

Appropriate care implies that the treatment should suit the patient. To investigate decision-making at the boundaries of palliative care we need to define the different phases of cancer care.

In the curative phase of care there is a realistic chance of cure or long lasting remission. The aim of care is survival of the patient. Ashby maintains that some harmful side effects of treatment may be acceptable to the patient for a good chance of cure.[1]

However, the term 'cure' may have different meanings for patients and professionals.

If a patient is to take an active part in decisions about his treatment he needs to have a clear idea of the goal of care. The patient may wonder if the treatment is going to prolong his life. If a treatment induces tumour shrinkage, a 'response', does it follow that quality of life improves?

Uncertainty for both patient and professional is a recurrent theme in the study. Professionals may exploit patients' misunderstandings about treatment goals:

> ...there would be some confusion in the patient's mind, we could well be exploiting that confusion as doctors, using it to defer any discussion on the matter.

This doctor admits that confusion about the aims of treatment might not be clarified to avoid having to explore potentially distressing issues about the progress of the cancer. This tactic is a form of distancing. Doctors are trained to cure diseases and may feel a sense of failure when confronted by a patient with advancing cancer which is no longer curable:

> I suppose we have it drummed in that we want to cure diseases and really what he was afraid of was having a big operation.

Some doctors may define a cure in terms of a five year disease-free survival.

> *I think it got to the point where she was discharged. That was the 5 years post-op and they said you needn't come anymore.*

For the patient, however, a 'cure ' is much more than survival for five years. It implies a return to the normality which existed before the onset of the cancer.[2]

The goals and aims of medical care often remain unclear to practitioners, patients and relatives. For instance, the process of referral to hospital may generate false hopes of a cure.

> *...you may think you've got the message across but unless you don't make any further referral the message doesn't sink in.*

> *I thought it was a difficult transitional phase, the curative to palliative. I found myself referring her back to the hospital clinic for further advice about this and looking back it was very inappropriate. I should have been looking at better palliation rather than back to the hospital.*

Again, a doctor admits that it is easier to refer to a hospital out-patient clinic, i.e. to be seen to be doing something active, than to consider whether further treatment is really going to improve the patient's quality of life.

Recurrence of cancer brings different problems since some patients may expect that there will always be some treatment available to keep the cancer at bay.

> *When he started getting problems with it later on that was hard, and it was hard for his wife as well because they thought he had got away with it.*

In some cases there is no curative phase of care and the aims of treatment are palliative from the outset:

> *It was very long drawn out, it was really palliative care from the word go.*

In other cases there may be a reluctance on the part of professionals to abandon active measures against the cancer:

> *Here was a letter which states, a long time before she died, when she developed meningeal involvement, that 'I'm afraid, no more chemotherapy is going to be any good here', and yet they kept on giving her intraspinal methotrexate after that.*

It may be difficult to know who should make the decision to cease chemotherapy. In this case the GP was frustrated because he did not understand why the patient was continuing to be offered chemotherapy.

Failure of cure in the context of life-threatening diseases presents particular difficulties for patients facing the unknown and for professionals who feel they may have failed.[17] There seems to be a particular pressure to continue treatment if the problem causing the patient's current deterioration is a direct result of previous medical treatment. For instance, when a patient developed a second malignancy as a consequence of previous therapy, doctors continued to advise further courses of treatment even when the chance of success was minimal.

This GP felt that ceasing active treatment should be a consultant decision:

> *I think it needed to be a hospital-based decision. Perhaps they should have sat down and said look there really is no*

> *point in doing this, that and the other, we really are treating*
> *symptoms. But she always faced you with a joyous expression:*
> *'OK, what can you do now?'*

The doctor acknowledges the difficulties facing hospital consultants in abandoning active therapies particularly when patients have expectations that there is always another treatment.

> *It would have been difficult to do that, in her case especially*
> *because she would have wanted you to do something else and*
> *expected you to do something else.*

It may be easier to offer another futile treatment than to spend time facing the reality of the situation.

> *I think that we probably go on pretending we can cure things*
> *unrealistically for longer than is justifiable.*

> *My biggest problem is what hospitals are doing to these*
> *patients and how much of that is truly palliative, how much*
> *is sticking your finger into the wind and saying, we'll try this*
> *next. A 'suck it and see' approach to palliative care. Now that*
> *worries me. I have concerns that that period of their life is*
> *made worse by suffering unnecessary exposure to therapy*
> *which causes problems..*

On the other hand, another GP did not experience difficulty in this area:

> *...a cure is not possible and they are not terminal, everything*
> *else is palliative.*

Although at a rational level a situation may be clearly palliative, the patient and physician may unconsciously push a goal approaching 'cure' rather than acknowledge palliation. It is possible that the reverse may occur, e.g. when patients with some forms of metastatic cancer are not treated when prolonged remission may be achievable.[17] A tension exists between a tendency to overtreat and overinvestigate and a fear of neglecting the patient.[34]

The transition to palliative care can be challenging for doctors as well as patients. Doctors may feel guilty that they did not act earlier:

> ...he had this peculiar pelvic pain which I never dreamt was likely to be related to what it was, we were thinking it was going to be musculo-skeletal or something very much more straightforward but it was the X-rays that revealed this deposit in his pelvis.

> But then in 1992 she developed this cough that didn't do as it should, it wasn't getting better and I can't remember how long I had been fiddling with it before we had a chest X-ray.

Many of the GPs identified difficulties because the patient had great resistance to accepting that the goal of care was palliative rather than curative. The doctor may feel more comfortable outlining what treatments are available than confronting difficult emotional issues surrounding death and dying.

> I could never say, 'there is nothing more I can do'. I think that's a ghastly way to say it to anybody, I think it's nicer to say 'well, no we can't cure that but we're going to do that, we're going to do this, we're going to make sure it's under control'.

There is indeed a great deal that can be done for a patient whose cancer is no longer curable. The patient should not be left feeling abandoned, but this is a point in the disease trajectory when it may be appropriate to assess the patient's needs. Some patients may initially cope by seeking further active treatments against the cancer:

> ...they kept asking for inappropriate things to be done because I don't think they had accepted that it was palliative.

Patients need to be aware that to feel fear and experience anxiety is part of the process of adjustment and they will need time with professionals that they trust to explore their fears.

> She had her X-ray which showed a pulmonary metastasis, and she was really quite devastated at that – then she knew she had got a cancer that had spread and she wanted any treatment that she could possibly have and she was always just a bit frightened when she talked about it – her voice would become slightly wobbly, she was frightened...

Although it is time-consuming and challenging to address the issues at the transition between cure and palliation it may make future care much more comfortable for patients and professionals if the patients are given time to come to terms with their situation.

> I think patients probably have to be given the permission to give up as well at times. They have to be offered have you had enough really, do you want to change tack from the way you're regarding this illness as something that you're going to overcome, to something that is eventually going to kill you? What do you want to do between now and then? I think that is probably a very difficult area for us – to make the switch from the pretence of cure to the acceptance that it is not going to and let's look at this in a different way. What are you going to do with your remaining months? I think one of the crucial hinge points is that change really. When the cards are on the table things are very much more open, it's very much easier.

Although this kind of communication with patients and relatives is difficult and time-consuming, once professionals and patients become partners and share common goals of care the whole situation is more relaxed. The alternative is to see some patients continuing with futile treatments. Doctors and nurses have an important role in helping patients to come to terms with their situation and to set realistic goals for the future.

A GP highlights the difficulties in changing from palliation to the terminal phase, but when the patient accepts this, care becomes easier.

> ...it is easier because everybody knows that there is nothing else that you can do except just be with the person.

Another GP explains how tensions may be eased once the decision about the aim of care is taken:

> Quite often I find when you have managed to get through the barrier it does become very much more relaxed for everybody.

> His final days were a lot easier really in terms of management than the time around the diagnosis, where there was the incredulity, disbelief...

Doctors may have difficulties in diagnosing when the terminal phase begins. The setting up of a syringe driver to deliver analgesics may be perceived as a medical last rite by professionals, patients and family.

> He said, I don't want to go on any longer, and that was when the syringe driver was started.

Some doctors see a patient taking to their bed as a sign of the terminal phase:

> I feel that once they get into bed they are terminal.

Others feel that the terminal phase starts when the patient 'gives up' and stops eating and drinking.

> When they appear to have given up I think, which they tend to do near the end, they don't want to eat, they don't want to drink anything, don't want to talk about anything and they tend to give up and want to die.

If there is a false hope that more active treatment is possible then patients may be admitted inappropriately and may have preferred to remain at home if they understood the reality of their situation:

> Now, I wonder if we'd managed to come to a more realistic consensus of her outlook whether that terminal admission would have been necessary. But we hadn't as yet come to a consensus between ourselves and she and her husband that she was that ill.

Admission to hospital may occur in the terminal phase as the stress becomes too much for the carers. Some patients and their families never reach acceptance and fight the disease to the end. In this case admission to hospital was seen as a sign that further treatment might be offered:

> I'm sure that they saw the admission to hospital, not as to provide palliative care but, you know, yet another last hope of can anything be done.

## Discussion

Nowadays, doctors may be concerned with applying a sophisticated technology to remove disease: the current concept of cure. Success may be measured in years of survival, not in terms of quality of life or freedom from sequelae of cancer or its treatment. In treatment of a cancer, a tumour response may or may not be translated into a survival advantage or better control of symptoms.[1] Iatrogenic side effects and illness implications may linger for months or years after a person experiences cancer treatment which has been medically defined as curative.[18]

For instance, in a study of 20 individuals pronounced cured, researchers found an enduring sense of vulnerability and evidence that reminders of their illness lingered.[19]

In another study, patients had lasting uncertainty, and fears of recurrence and of a second malignancy.[20] Andersen quotes 20% of cancer survivors experiencing significant psychological adjustment difficulties.[21] Even when adverse effects of treatment or the underlying disease do not occur the patient with cancer may remain preoccupied with his/her health. This preoccupation may take the form of nagging health worries or anxieties about death.[21]

In summary, it appears that the patient's perception of cure is related to his illness, whilst the doctor's is centred on the disease. In our quest for the certainty of clinical cure we risk failing to understand the meaning of the experience of cancer for the patient. The patient needs an explanation for their illness that connects their personal experience to their broader, culturally defined interpretation. For a patient with cancer, 'cure' is not therefore the end point, but the beginning of a time of struggle when healthcare support is likely to be withdrawn.[2]

In palliative care, the aim of treatment is to maximise the patient's quality of life. The transition between a curative and a palliative approach can be filled with uncertainty. The doctor or nurse may feel, or even say, 'There is nothing more I can do'.[22]

In the cancer context, clinicians offer differing definitions of the starting point of palliative care. Calman states that palliative care begins when the diagnosis of cancer is established, death is certain and likely in the near future, and a curative approach to care has been abandoned.[23]

This statement does not help us in deciding when to abandon a curative approach. It also seems to exclude situations where 'aggressive' chemotherapy is given with apparent curative intent to patients with widespread cancer.

Doctors may, however, be placed in a difficult situation by relatives who equate continuing active treatment with maintaining the patient's hope and morale.[2] These attitudes are one consequence of the medicalisation of death. Many think that acknowledging death may cause the patient to give up. The situation is compounded by myths that morphine hastens death and the prejudice of those committed to the curative model of medical care. The notions that all treatment is good medicine, or that hope and treatment are the same thing are common. These ideas may be a consequence of our society's unfamiliarity with death. Dying is often perceived to be a frightening, painful process which should occur in hospital, rather than at home.

In the terminal stage, the patient's condition leaves no room for doubt that death is near and likely to occur within a matter of days.[24] The patient is profoundly weak, bed-bound, drowsy, disorientated in time and has a severely limited attention span, is increasingly disinterested in food and drink and is finding it difficult to swallow medication.[24]

When in the terminal phase of illness, all unnecessary treatments are withdrawn and 'no treatment related side effects are acceptable'.[1]

The dilemma for a professional is when to continue to strive to prolong an individual patient's life and when to focus care on the patient's quality of life and cease active therapies: the dilemma of care versus cure.[25] Professionals then need to cope with an uncertainty which appears to relate not so much to the need for palliation but to the timing of it in the spectrum of care.[26] Patients and their families also need to know what the term 'palliation' means, so that they have a clear idea of the goals of care and the resources available to support them.[27] A clear concept of palliative care may give professional carers permission to address these issues with patients while active treatment is still being attempted.[28] In attempting to acknowledge the patient as a person first, the palliative care worker is exposed to the stresses of resolving ethical dilemmas and dealing with his/her own pain and grief.

A smooth transition between curative, palliative and terminal phases of care is facilitated by facing the issues of death and dying. Death-denying attitudes with unrealistic expectations of medicine from patients, relatives and doctors are sources of distress for patients with incurable cancer.[1]

# CHAPTER THREE

# PALLIATIVE CHEMOTHERAPY
# AND QUALITY OF LIFE

*The old men ask
For more time, while the young
Waste it. And the philosopher
Smiles, knowing there is none.*

**R S Thomas**

Chemotherapy, radiotherapy and surgery may be used in a palliative context to improve quality of life by relieving distressing symptoms and to prolong survival.[29,30] A dilemma for the clinician is to balance the possible benefits of the intervention against the risks of side effects which may reduce the patient's quality of life.

Some GPs felt that lack of time was an important factor influencing oncologists to continue with chemotherapy in patients with advancing disease. Prescribing chemotherapy may be an easier option, in a busy clinic, than discussing stopping active treatments.

> *I think oncology out-patient clinics have become horrendously busy... one suspects that at times it's probably easier to try something else rather than to sit down and discuss it.*

Chemotherapy is often given with palliative intent. It is therefore important to assess the effect of chemotherapy on quality of life, and whether it actually does relieve symptoms i.e. palliates. There are patients with extensive disease who do not have any symptoms. It is difficult to make these patients feel better with active treatment.[31] There is a widespread tendency to underestimate the toxicity of treatment.[34]

> *...she was having this chemo that made her feel absolutely terrible. I remember thinking I wasn't sure the chemo was doing her any good but I felt I ought to encourage her to take it even though her quality of life was hopeless on it.*

Doctors sometimes have an urge to 'do something' and this may lead to inappropriate use of drugs or chemotherapy:

> *...you could say to them now we've tried this and this and it hasn't been very good but there are one or two other things we can try...*

These examples question the motives for continuing chemotherapy in advanced cancer. There are doubts in some GPs' minds as to the benefit of this form of treatment to improve quality of life. There was a feeling amongst some doctors that whilst palliative radiotherapy relieved symptoms, chemotherapy did not.

> *I think there is a vast difference between chemotherapy and palliative radiotherapy which, in general, is effective short term in relieving bone pain and doesn't make one feel that bad.*

> *I think the radiotherapy was a genuine attempt to palliate and relieve symptoms but I can't quite see why they went on giving her intravenous drugs, not after they had already decided it would seem that there wasn't any point in giving her more.*

Side effects from treatment were severe in some cases:

> *...she had lots of chemotherapy into her hand and she had a necrotic ulcer on her hand and that actually caused everybody far more angst than her real illness.*

> *It was a struggle going back to hospital for chemotherapy, that's the distance, it was an effort, she did feel very ill.*

The impact on a patient's quality of life of travel to a clinic to have chemotherapy is often disregarded in weighing the benefits and harms of treatment.

The futility of some forms of treatment also causes distress to professionals.

> *Many of the drugs that they are giving are dreadfully toxic. I have got a woman at the moment with carcinoma of the breast with secondaries, it's very painful and disfiguring, and*

*they are giving her very aggressive chemotherapy at the moment which is making her dreadfully ill, she vomits profusely and feels absolutely awful, and she has had three lots which haven't made the slightest difference so far to her tumour... I felt well, really is it worth pursuing making her life even worse? I feel somehow that the medical profession may have failed her, but I don't know.*

However the problem for oncologists in decision-making is that there are occasional patients who improve dramatically with active treatments. It is not possible at present to predict which patients will respond well. The GP acknowledges uncertainty about this view since some patients do benefit from palliative chemotherapy:

*Having said that, over the last two or three years, I have been surprised by advances in oncology and their ability to produce a remission. I think I was right in my opinion more ten years ago than I am now because they have made some advances in that area.*

Another doctor describes the uncertainty in this area of care, in a case in which the patient did live much longer than he expected and where active treatment did confer benefits to the patient's quality of life.

*She was miserable and she lost all her hair, she had nasty chemo side effects and that took up the first couple of months really, the sort of morale boosting. But then once we had got her anti-emetics right and the chemotherapy off and her wig she was very happy and she had a lovely Christmas.*

Perhaps it is the occasional individual case which responds dramatically well to active treatments that drives some doctors to continue with heroic treatments for patients in the face of advancing disease.

Chemotherapy is sometimes used as a way of offering hope in an otherwise desperate situation. But, since this form of treatment carries such a risk of toxicity and does little to meet patients' real needs for honest, sensitive communication, it should not be used to give false hope.

> It would always be, well I'm seeing him again in a fortnight's time, this doesn't seem to be working and I hope he'll change it to something better. It's very difficult to knock someone if the seeds of doubt haven't been sown by the consultant.

> I don't think she actually said to them, I want to go on being treated, but I think the patient expectation that she should continue to receive care and attention and treatment from them must have been there.

> I think that they find it very difficult to divorce the fact that they are going to the clinic from the fact that there must be some hope somewhere, so that their mind is slightly twisted towards, well they wouldn't be doing all this just for another couple of months of life, there must be some hope somewhere.

> If somebody wants to still go up there and wants treatment it's very difficult to refuse people their last hope but it's probably a very expensive way of doing it and probably not the best way of doing it.

These comments highlight the doctors' anxieties about whether it is ethical to give palliative chemotherapy as a way of maintaining hope. It seems that patients assume that they must have a good chance of prolonged survival if they are going through this demanding form of therapy. By persisting with therapy, consultants may be generating false hopes of recovery. At times it may be the GP who generates false hope:

*I think that we'd rather collude with them because... one might find oneself saying, we can't cure it but we're trying to stop it progressing, which is a very sort of fuzzy thing to say really but it gives them a little bit of hope and it's a comfortable thing for us to say.*

This doctor is honestly admitting that saying that further active treatment would be futile is difficult. Perhaps if palliative care was perceived as a treatment rather than as part of 'giving up' then professionals might feel more comfortable at this stage of the disease.

Valuable time may be spent in pursuing treatments which are futile as a form of bargaining between doctor and patient.

*He wanted to feel that the specialist still had something up his sleeve but I think he knew really that he was quite near the end. But again, all the way through we had this problem of, there was always going to be some offer of treatment and there never seemed to be a point where you could actually say to them no, there isn't any more treatment, our aim should be to make you as comfortable as possible, you don't need to worry about any pain, everything will be done to make everything as pleasant as we possibly can. You could never have a conversation which wasn't geared to treatment.*

It seems that the most difficult issue for doctors is the conversation around the issue of the fact that there is no further active treatment option.

On the other hand, bargaining may be an essential part of helping a patient to come to terms with their situation:

*I've not had anybody yet saying they would like to live the maximum regardless of suffering, and a very large number would say to you straight away that they would be very glad if you just saw them off.*

The issue of active chemotherapy at the end of life remains a concern for many of the doctors although this doctor agrees that it may be ethical to give chemotherapy as a means of preserving hope.

*If people like to feel that they are still fighting then I don't see all that much harm in regimes that aren't going to be accompanied by too much ill-health really, I feel more strongly about things that are going to wipe people out, make them sick, make them feel dreadful, detract significantly from what quality of life they have left, chasing a 5% chance of response.*

Giving a treatment may be a way of avoiding difficult communication issues.

*I think he'd given up then and knew that nothing else could be done and they were flapping around trying to get something done all the time. I think he'd actually accepted it for definite and they still didn't want to accept it and they kept asking for things to be done.*

Oncologists sometimes seem to continue treatment inappropriately.

*I have known him frequently say to people, my advice to you is to have none, not to even start, I don't think we've got anything useful to offer. He is quite prepared to do that, he is quite prepared to stand up and be counted. It isn't an easy option to tell someone no, I recognise that and he is quite prepared to do that, but once he has started, he doesn't seem to know when to stop. He seems to quite often continue when it does seem to be hopeless.*

This observation suggests that, just as in other areas of medical care, withdrawing therapy may present more of a problem for oncologists than not starting it. One doctor suggests that a team approach may lead to better decision-making:

> I think that they need to have a discussion before they decide and I don't see how that could be done very easily. To be honest, I think that you almost need a case conference type of approach.

Doctors and patients have different ways of coping with these difficulties. Some adopt an optimistic approach:

> He was really given the impression that if he suffered slightly unpleasant treatment from time to time that he would go on living for years. And right from the beginning that appeared to me to be incredibly optimistic.

But some GPs felt that the blame for inappropriate treatment should not be laid at the oncologist's door:

> I think that the solution is probably, the patient wouldn't get the chemotherapy if we didn't send them up there. I think there are at least two areas; one is for us to have the knowledge and the confidence to say no, enough is enough.

This acknowledges that just mentioning referral to the oncologist may lead the patient to believe that further active treatments are available to help him.

> I think the other thing is sufficient skill in terms of talking to people with terminal illnesses and talking about things that are uncomfortable...

This highlights the need for improved communication skills. Doctors need to learn how to talk to patients about ceasing treatment of the cancer without causing the patient to lose hope.

> *It's easy to hide behind the fact that she wanted to go on, but perhaps they didn't give her enough opportunities to stop by being skilful enough to broach the self-evident fact that she wasn't getting any better and in fact getting worse really.*

Some GPs felt they were left out of decisions once the patient went to hospital:

> *I thought I was peripheral in what was going on at this stage...*

> *I can fairly say, without wishing to pass the buck, that what was going on wasn't something that I could follow as a general practitioner. Her various forms of therapy and her clinical state were such that I didn't know whether there was sense in it or no sense.*

It was difficult for some GPs to let their consultant colleagues know of their reservations about treatment decisions.

> *I wasn't involved in the decision at all. It was something that the patient accepted quite readily and therefore I didn't really feel there was any point in my intervening.*

Other GPs felt that they were well informed by hospital staff:

> *I didn't really find it objectionable and they were quite good about ringing me up.*

This GP would have liked to be involved in the decision-making process:

*It's actually very difficult to talk to people [consultants] who
have actually made a decision, you see they don't talk to you
in General Practice at a time when they are about to make a
decision. In fact, they don't talk to you about their decisions,
they make a decision and then you're left carrying the can
often as a GP. At which point it is very difficult for you to
change the direction of the treatment.*

An ethical problem arises when the autonomy of the patient conflicts
with that of a close relative, for instance in the question of whether to
continue with chemotherapy:

*...she had an informed choice to stop it but her husband was
always very keen for her to continue because he wanted her to
have all the treatment that could be given for her.*

It may be that, like some doctors and nurses, relatives find it difficult
to abandon active therapies.

*That's the major part, they don't want to be seen to be giving
up, they want to be seen to be trying to think of something
new to get them better. If you sit back and do nothing it looks
as if you've given up almost.*

## Discussion

Inappropriate treatments may cause harm in a number of ways.
Physical suffering may result from the side effects of such treatment,
e.g. hair loss and vomiting from chemotherapy. Distress may also be
caused by raising false hopes in the patient and family. Such
inappropriate treatment encourages patients, relatives and doctors to
avoid the reality of death. Instead, time should be spent helping the
patient to come to terms with her death and to complete 'unfinished

business'. On a wider scale, the inappropriate use of expensive treatments is wasteful of limited medical resources which might have been used to benefit other patients.

There is often great uncertainty in predicting the outcome of an intervention in an individual case, to which may be added the uncertainties of predicting the prognosis. The decision of whether to give treatment requires the informed consent of the patient who needs to be aware of his choices, including that of best supportive palliative care.

Slevin et al. compared the responses of patients with cancer with those of a matched control group, cancer specialists, general practitioners and cancer nurses in assessing personal cost-benefit of chemotherapy. In their study, most patients were willing to accept intensive chemotherapy for a very small chance of benefit, in contrast to healthy controls or to the choices made by healthcare professionals.[32] Increased participation in decision-making means that patients need more information about their disease and treatment options. People with cancer find it difficult to accept circumstances in which there are no active treatments directed against the cancer. The wish of the patient to have treatment in the face of little prospect of benefit presents an ethical dilemma for the doctor.

Slevin et al. reported that patients with cancer were much more likely to opt for chemotherapy with minimal chance of benefit than were their professional carers and people without cancer.[32] They also found attitudes changed drastically once cancer had been diagnosed. Patients were more likely to accept investigations and invasive procedures than were nurses. The authors concluded that care must be taken to ensure that judgements and attitudes of staff are not denying patients simple tests or interventions from which they may derive benefit.[32,33]

Some patients are happy for the doctor to advise them what to do. This may be a problem if we adhere too rigidly to the doctrine of respect for patient autonomy at all times. Such respect for autonomy needs to be flexible enough to allow patients the choice of leaving the decision about the best course of action to the doctor if they wish. Such a voluntary surrender of autonomy is not paternalism. Taking responsibility for his choices may mean that the patient will blame himself if events turn out badly.

The majority of chemotherapy is given with palliative intent.[34] A rational use of cytotoxic drugs involves a trade-off between likely benefits and expected side effects. The use of potentially lethal treatments needs to be justified by the likelihood of prolonged remissions or that there will be such a regression of the cancer as to result in an improved quality of life for the patient.[34] There is a risk of overestimating the value of chemotherapy and undervaluing the impact of toxicity on quality of life.[34] The proliferation of intensive investigations puts the clinician under further pressure to do something.[34] It may also be easier to prescribe an active treatment than to confront the difficult issues of death and dying.[34] Much scepticism exists about partial responses which may misrepresent the impact of chemotherapy. Even if one accepts the difficulties in measuring and assessing the partial response it does not necessarily correlate with relief of symptoms, improved quality of life or useful expression of life.[34] We need empirical information about the probabilities of harms and benefits that may occur as a result of medical interventions.[35]

We need to find out what patients think and help them make decisions about treatment. The dialogue this demands is challenging because it threatens the adaptive suppression that many patients use to protect themselves from negative feelings. Unfortunately, the consequence of avoiding this dialogue is unnecessary treatment given with misunderstood intentions.[36]

There is no standard quality of life measure for use in palliative care. The current quality of life scales each measure differing aspects of the patient's life. A questionnaire needs to be relevant and brief; they are generally less useful than in-depth interviews in obtaining accurate quality of life data.

Sheldon highlights the difficulties in making decisions because patients, like everyone, are inconsistent.[37] Their responses to decisions about treatment may be different when discussed with oncologists or with palliative care teams. Different disciplines need to maintain clear channels of communication to acknowledge these difficulties and to reach a consensus rather than perceiving one discipline as being critical of another.

# CHAPTER FOUR

# DIFFICULTIES IN
# COMMUNICATING
# WITH PATIENTS

*What moment worse*
*Than that young doctor trying to explain?*

Douglas Dunn

## Breaking bad news

Honest communication is essential if patients, their families and doctors are to share common aims of treatment. The relationship between doctor and patient lies at the core of clinical medicine. It is a relationship based on mutual trust. The uncertainty imposed on this relationship by a diagnosis of incurable cancer generated difficulties for the general practitioners.

> *I would like to have a good conversation along those lines with, say, 80% of my palliative care patients but I probably manage it with closer to 50%.*

Doctors often had close relationships with their patients prior to the diagnosis of cancer. A young doctor highlighted the importance of a good doctor-patient relationship and felt that her youth was perhaps a disadvantage.

> *When you don't have a personal relationship with somebody who gets ill it's a bit of a problem and also my relative youth.*

A GP generally knows his/her patients, but this may be a disadvantage at times.

> *...you tend to see people in a certain context and he was somebody that we saw a lot anyway with largely psychiatric or psychological problems so people tend to get pigeon-holed.*

Doctors often expressed feelings of guilt at the time of diagnosis and may compensate for this by being over attentive in future.

> *I missed the diagnosis in the first place, well I was slow picking up on it, and I do actually wonder if that was influencing me very much in going along with everything that this family wanted.*

One reason why professionals find breaking bad news so difficult is that they fear the patient will blame them. Historically, the bearer of bad tidings has been identified with the message he carries. Delaying treatment is also a common cause of guilt amongst the doctors.

> *...whenever you eventually make the diagnosis, or it is made, you look back and think, did I make it soon enough or was it something that has been staring me in the face for six months that I've not picked up?*

Cancer often presents with vague symptoms so time passes before specific symptoms and signs of serious disease develop. Doctors who have acted in a paternalistic fashion in the earliest stages of the disease, by giving inappropriate reassurance or refusing a patient's request for further investigations, are especially liable to be blamed for the bad news when it emerges later.

Patients may accept their situation and face their own deaths in a calm way. A strong faith may help some to cope with uncertainty.

> *She was an extremely religious person and a very committed Christian, and had absolutely no doubt in her mind of an after-life.*

On the other hand, communication and care may both be more difficult if the patient denies the reality of the situation. The doctor may feel he has not given the best care:

> *Because she refused to acknowledge the situation it was very difficult to talk.*

Patients may react by denying the diagnosis and this can make further care difficult for the doctor:

*...she then refused a mastectomy and refused I think in a*
*way, to actually come to terms with it and her way of dealing*
*with that was to withdraw into herself.*

Denial acts as a buffer against unexpected shocking news, allowing the patient time to prepare himself. In this situation, denial acts as a useful coping strategy. Nevertheless, the same patient may be willing to talk about the diagnosis and prognosis at a later stage.

People have differing coping strategies and it is interesting to note that doctors may feel uncomfortable if patients employ distancing tactics, just as patients complain about doctors who distance themselves:

*...you felt you were kept at such a distance, that there were*
*lots of things that one could do to help but you weren't*
*allowed to.*

Deafness and language difficulties challenge communication skills. It may be difficult for the GP to see the patient on his own and the consultation becomes a family meeting in which different family members have differing needs which may be difficult to address in a group situation.

*He didn't talk about it very much at all and didn't want to.*
*His wife did but he showed it in different ways, he got very*
*tearful and low but really didn't want to talk about it much.*
*It was difficult because his family was always there, his sons,*
*and always something had got to be done.*

Doctors have many different ways of reacting to the uncertainty of the situation. Some fear the unknown:

*I don't know, because by exploring it we might have opened a*
*can of worms really...*

Some feel that a patient would be shocked if a doctor explored their feelings about their illness and their future:

> *You're not too sure what is going on in their mind and are quite happy for it to remain that way, that uncertainty. It would require the agenda to be set by the patient before you would raise it, for fear of adding to their uncertainty.*

Others feel that it is right to follow the patient's agenda:

> *I think that you should try and be what they want you to be because at the end of the day it's their death and their relatives and their family.*

> *I think, had she ever said to me, do you think it's worth it, I would have said no, but she never really wanted to hear that, she never wanted to hear anyone saying we'd give up.*

## Giving the prognosis

The prognosis is usually uncertain. A patient may look as though he will live only hours and in fact survive for days.[24]

> *This chap went on for months and I thought he was going to die long before he did, some people seem to hang on, but as I say it is difficult to tell, it almost takes you by surprise.*

> *The prognostic problem is that we have often got a greater uncertainty, even when you know exactly what's wrong with somebody, the physical signs and symptoms that tell you the rate at which somebody is declining are very poor at prediction.*

Doctors may fear the harm they may cause:

> *You always have the fear that you are going to unnecessarily upset the patient.*

> *You don't want to tell them how dreadful some end points can*
> *be and it all sounds so frightening.*

Generally the doctors wanted to be honest but found this area difficult because of their genuine uncertainty as to how the disease would progress:

> *...because translating that academic information into*
> *specific cases is something that you can't do and the*
> *consultant, he can do it with honesty because he is dealing*
> *with populations, we deal with people, individuals.*

Patients, however, need information, though each individual has differing needs. Some wish to know everything and others wish to leave this area to the doctor.

> *I was never more than one reference of the text books ahead of*
> *him really in terms of my knowledge of this, how it was likely*
> *to respond, what was likely to be suggested, so that was a bit*
> *uncomfortable really.*

> *She did ask questions and she clearly wanted to be told the*
> *truth and no one I think, certainly not me, tried to pull the*
> *wool over her eyes as far as the prognosis was concerned.*

Many doctors felt that the patient intuitively knew the situation.

> *I don't think there was any discussion with him about his*
> *future but I think he... there was a look... he looked back at*
> *you steadily. You know, we don't need to spell this out but I*
> *know, my impression was that he was aware.*

> *He preferred to cope, I think, with dealing with individual*
> *symptoms as they arose but I don't think there is any doubt*
> *that he knew that his life expectancy was very much curtailed*
> *by this but we didn't ever have the conversation.*

*I think that they may have asked then, but I think nearer the end they actually knew. They came to terms with it at the very last minute, just before he died really. I don't ever remember them really asking, because that's difficult as well if anybody asks because you can never tell really can you?*

*I always try and encourage people, indirectly in her instance, to go and have their holidays and to enjoy life but without saying enjoy it while you can. You imply that in a way, don't you.*

Others take a pessimistic view:

*I think you have to be very vague and explain the difficulty that you can't tell and I think you have to be pessimistic rather than optimistic.*

This doctor manages the uncertainty by acknowledging its existence:

*I always preface whatever I say by, I'm always hopeless about getting it right. I think it's bloody difficult for anybody to get it right.*

Part of the difficulty for professionals is that they feel a burden of expectation from the patient and relatives.

*I think you have to tell them you don't know and that nobody knows because again they'll blame you, well not blame you but they don't want to hear that, because they expect you to know everything.*

Others feel the best approach is to explore the future with the patient.

*I usually ask why, what event is it that they are looking towards and try and give them some ideas. I generally don't*

*try and pin myself down because it is very difficult, they start
ticking the months off on the calendar.*

For some it is the practical issues of living which precipitate
discussion about prognosis.

*I said look, I think if you are going to sell this property
you've really got to get on with it because... you know... I
find talking about prognosis... I find it terribly difficult to
be good about prognosis and I'm hopeless at it really.*

*I remember a poor man who was dying of a carcinoma of the
prostate, who suddenly became dreadfully poorly with
hypercalcaemia and was obviously going to die in a matter of
days and I was telling his wife who said, 'Oh my God, he
hasn't made a will'.*

Some doctors felt it was best to talk in general terms:

*I try to give the patient as full an understanding as I can of
the situation...*

Some are guided by what they would wish for themselves:

*I really don't think, if I'm dying of something, I don't want
to know what's going on.*

There is a feeling that the level of information given should be
tailored to the needs of the patient.

*I do feel you have got to try to feel your way, to try and
understand what the patient really wants to know.*

Patients react to a poor prognosis in differing ways.

*I'm sure I shy away from saying that sort of thing sometimes because you just don't want the pain and agony of saying it all and because it's difficult to say it, and you know they're going to go away and their life will feel shattered for days.*

Doctors, patients and relatives find talking about prognosis stressful. Doctors may feel a real sense of failure.

*We have had people who have burst into tears and become hysterical but not very often... more likely it would be a relative that would do that. Often the patient says 'I know', that's more often the case. I suppose it's also the doctor giving up on the patient really, and you've got to accept that you're giving up.*

Choosing the appropriate language is important.

*They needed it spelling out to them but I find that very difficult to do because it appears that you are hard and don't care, doesn't it.*

Patients may react with a fighting spirit:

*Some people cling on to life in such a way that makes you wonder if you haven't done your job properly in maybe the first instance, they are so frightened of death.*

There have been suggestions that those patients with a fighting spirit live longer than those who give up.[103] Greater patient symptom distress has been associated with a shorter prognosis.[38,39,40]

Others deal with distressing news by denial, which may be an effective coping mechanism for the patient but leaves the doctor feeling uncomfortable.

## Discussion

The question of length of life remaining to the patient is important for many different reasons. The patient may have unfinished business, goals to achieve, or wish to spend time with their family. Relatives, too, often want to know what is going to happen and may wish to be present at the death.[41] Information about the likely prognosis is indispensable for the doctor in determining whether to continue active treatments with a potential for harm. An accurate estimate of survival would allow professionals to plan the ideal therapeutic strategy between overtreatment and neglect, to answer questions from patient and family, and to organise help for the patient.[42]

Predicting when death is going to occur may be difficult.[43,44,45] Specialist palliative care nurses and hospice units emphasise the importance of early referral of patients, if the highest standards of care are to be achieved. On the other hand, general practitioners are often faced with uncertainty about the rate of progress of the disease and defer referral to such specialists until 'the end'.

Talking about a poor prognosis may be even more difficult than giving a diagnosis of cancer. The doctors experienced great uncertainty and believed that there were no reliable prognostic indicators, nor did they feel that any other professional was any better at judging the likely length of survival of an individual patient. A patient may look as though he will only live for few hours but then survive for several days.[24]

Doctors tend to overestimate the length of survival.[43,44,46,47] It is possible that accuracy is improved with increasing clinical experience.[48,49]

The findings from these interviews are supported by past research. No professional group is better than another when it comes to predicting the survival of an individual patient.[43,44,46,50] Patient gender, marital status, age, pain score, knowledge of diagnosis or number of drugs prescribed do not predict prognosis. Nor is there a direct association between functional status and prognosis.[48] Weakness and immobility may be prognostic factors but quality of life is not.[51,52] There is however a suggestion that quality of life indices may have a predictive value in patients with advanced breast cancer having chemotherapy.[53]

Nutritional status seems to be an important prognostic factor, with poor nutritional status and a low serum albumen being predictive of a poor prognosis.[54,55,56] Raised bilirubin, low performance status, hypotension, and requirement for admission at first referral to specialist palliative care, predicted for poor survival.[57] Cognitive failure and psychological issues are controversial.[58] Perhaps further research needs to be conducted to explore what patients feel about their own life expectancy.[41]

The uncertainties experienced in the scenario of breaking bad news are heightened when trying to communicate a poor prognosis. This uncertainty makes it difficult for doctors to decide when to stop actively trying to treat the cancer.

## Maximising choice

When considering the management of a patient with advanced cancer, factors such as length of survival and quality of life need careful consideration by patients, relatives and professionals. Quality of life is difficult to define because it is a dynamic concept which changes with time and has a large subjective component.[59] For patients with advanced cancer, good health is not possible but other factors are important in maintaining a good quality of life, including physical, psychological, social and spiritual issues. Thus, quality of life relates to objective features of the disease and side effects of treatment but also to subjective feelings and to the patient's hopes.[60] The concept of quality of life extends to respect the autonomy of the patient in body, mind and spirit in the context of social relationships with others.[22]

In expressing his/her autonomy, an individual shapes and gives meaning to their life. Autonomy may be defined as the capacity to think, decide and act on the basis of such thought and decision, freely and independently.[61] In a situation where death is, or is thought to be, imminent, then respect for another's autonomy assumes a particular importance. Patients with advanced cancer can appear physically frail and are vulnerable to well-intentioned medical intervention or paternalism.

Paternalism is a denial of autonomy and a substitution of an individual's choices for his own good.[62] Patient autonomy can be protected from paternalistic intervention by a strict requirement for informed consent. The central function of informed consent is to ensure a sharing of power between patient and doctor.

Calman has developed a useful way of looking at quality of life issues.[23] He suggests that the quality of life measures the difference, or gap, between the hopes and expectations of the individual and that individual's present experiences or reality.[23] A good quality of life can be said to exist when an individual's hopes are matched by the reality of his experience, i.e. when the gap is small. The opposite is also true; when there is a large gap between hopes and reality the quality of life is low. To improve quality of life we need to reduce the gap between hopes and reality and to help people achieve realistic goals.

A GP gives a good description of a patient exercising control and his autonomous choice to make the most of his remaining life:

*Now, if you talked to that man a month or two before he died, he would say quite openly, the last six months of my life are by far the happiest of my life. It was the most incredible atmosphere in that house when you went there, every evening, it was almost a non-stop party...*

Patients need to have the opportunity to make their own choices regarding treatment and their place of death. They may be frightened of being a burden to their family.

*...each separate patient needs a very individual package.*

The choice of the place of death is important:

*What he didn't want, but unfortunately had to happen in the end, was to go into hospital. He wanted to stay at home as long as possible, to live independently as long as possible.*

*I got the distinct impression that she wanted to stay at home.*

The proportion of people dying at home as compared to hospital is currently dropping by 1% each year. Patients still spend 90% of the last year of life at home. Specialist palliative home care teams do enable patients to remain at home longer.[63] In a study of 94 patients, 58% wanted to die at home, 20% in hospital, 20% in a hospice and 2% elsewhere.[64]

Of the patients who did die at home, 94% had expressed a preference for this, but of those dying in hospital, 69% had stated an alternative preference.

Cartwright's survey of general practitioners, hospital consultants, community nurses and relatives revealed that all these groups wanted more people to be looked after in their own homes rather than die in hospital if adequate care could be arranged at home.[65]

Thorpe[104] has suggested that to enable dying people to remain at home they need:

- adequate nursing care
- a night sitting service
- good symptom control
- confident and committed GPs
- access to specialist palliative care
- effective co-ordination of care
- financial support
- terminal care education.

Patients have a need to be in control, to exert their autonomy and to reflect on their decisions.

Patients may exercise their autonomy by choosing alternative therapies:

> *If somebody wishes to treat themselves when we can't help*
> *them anyway, I don't worry. I find it much more frustrating if*
> *there's good medical treatment for something, I then do find*
> *it difficult sometimes.*

To make autonomous choices there is a need for honest information given at a pace at which the patient can comprehend what is happening.

> *I think one of the difficulties in this case was the fact that he*
> *was a particular introspective individual who liked to be kept*
> *in the picture as much as possible.*

These conversations necessarily require time from the doctor. Patients still want an opportunity to discuss issues of treatment choices with a doctor. In the constrained healthcare system in which we operate these discussions may be delegated to nurses.

It may be difficult if different professionals are giving different messages.

> *I do find that helpful, that it's the specialist's policy to be honest with people... people don't come back with some vague story of ulcers and inflammation and things that you eventually have to unravel and put right.*

Being optimistic in a situation where the prognosis is likely to be poor may be easier for the professional in the short term. However, someone will be faced with the problems of an angry patient and relative when it becomes apparent that the disease is progressing.

> *I think people just aren't honest enough and they tend to give an optimistic view. I can remember someone in exactly the same situation as you and we did this, that and the other and I saw them last week and they still were at the bowling club... and this was three years ago they were in the same situation as you now... They're the best that can possibly happen, we don't say the 95% that doesn't happen to. So, it's good at the time, it's easy at the time but it doesn't help in the long term.*

Such an over-optimistic policy can have sad consequences for the patient.

> *I think now people give a rather optimistic view of things and when things don't turn out like that they start to lose faith. Perhaps if we were pessimistic about how things were everything would be a bonus.*

Weakness from advanced cancer can impair the physical autonomy to move around.

> Her quality of life was fairly poor. She spent a lot of time in bed. I wasn't sure why she spent so much time in bed, I thought she was well enough to get up but that seemed to be the role of the person that was sick.

Physical weakness may tempt the doctor to feel he has to act paternalistically.

> She was tiny to start with and then of course became tinier and tinier. She was the sort of person you could feel very protective of really because she was very frail.

Quality of life data are little used in decision-making in oncology practice. There is a need to inform clinical decision-making with quality of life data which relate to patient orientated rather than tumour related outcomes.[66]

Respect for patient autonomy demands that patients be given honest answers to their questions. Without honesty, moral discourse becomes impossible and communication pointless. Without honest information, a patient becomes more uncertain and is unable to make decisions about his future. Patients need just as much information to make rational decisions about their medical condition as they do for any other sphere of their lives.

## How to introduce specialist palliative care

GPs wanted to involve specialist palliative care nurses at an early stage although they feared what the patient might think.

> I tend to involve the nurses at a very early stage. I look for an

> *excuse to get the nurses in to make a relationship with somebody who is having difficulties of a nursing nature.*

Specialist palliative care services have a clearer role in supporting the primary healthcare team.

> *I think there was a time when the role of the hospice was probably not well understood by District Nurses but I don't think there was any problem here.*

However, some GPs rightly felt that not all dying patients need specialist palliative care.

> *If there is a good family support then our District Nurse, the GP and the family are sufficient and they don't want 'outsiders'.*

Specialist palliative care can support and complement the primary care team.

> *I'm always keen to have them in there as early as possible. I also find that a bit difficult, I find myself saying there is a specialist team that are very good at helping and supporting people with long term illness and I always find myself saying, it's not just cancer.*

# CHAPTER FIVE

# RELIEF OF PAIN
# AND SUFFERING

*The angels of morphia have borne him up*

**Sylvia Plath**

## Pain and symptom control

A fundamental aim of palliative care is to control pain and other distressing symptoms which impair a patient's quality of life. Difficulties were frequently reported in controlling pain.

> *I felt that we never really got on top of her bone pain.*

Some ethical dilemmas caused the doctors great distress and led some to question the prolongation of the dying process.

> *When she came back with the syringe driver in she looked awful and she was awful, we had a hell of job controlling her pain and at one point her dose of diamorphine was going up and up and up to enormous levels, we weren't really winning… I thought, what are we going to do about this woman's pain, I was almost at the point of despair what to do next…*

Fears about using morphine are not confined to patients. Some doctors expressed concerns, as did some relatives:

> *I've seen somebody who was on so much morphine she was toxic and twitching and I've been very cautious of it since. I always feel badly if they are obviously have tiny little pupils and feel dopey and zonked out, that's not right either.*

> *I think that badly affected her quality of life for the last year or so really. The daughter said, 'No, that's an opiate, that'll kill you'.*

Several GPs felt that the terminal phase needed to be fairly short, that there was a pressure to avoid a lingering death.

> *My feeling, I suppose, is that the length of time that somebody is terminally ill should be as short as possible. I think the*

*stress of it, certainly for the carers and relatives, the shorter a
timespan of terminal illness the better.*

Anxieties are expressed about the ethical issues involved in giving
adequate doses of analgesics which might also have an effect of
shortening life.

> *I think one of my lessons that I have learnt is, not to, I almost
> sort of feel that you don't let people off the hook, once they
> have reached the point of becoming terminal rather than
> palliative, the worst thing, I think, is having to go through the
> agony of letting go twice.*

A prolonged dying process is stressful for all concerned. The patient
here is clinging to the hope of recovery.

> *I think I found it uncomfortable because she was so
> frightened. We did discuss the cancer but not actually the
> dying side of it. I think I was always ending up trying to
> reassure her because she would say, oh, that doesn't mean
> that it's spread there does it...*

In some cases patient may request euthanasia:

> *I think certainly looking after somebody who is dying of
> protracted malignancy, when you reach the point where you
> feel their quality of life is so bloody awful that they actually
> say to you their quality of life is awful and they don't want
> to go on, sometimes they do say that to you, they really don't
> want to go on, they want as little a time as possible please,
> and sometimes they even ask you to finish them off. Now a lot
> of them actually really do mean it, a lot of them don't of
> course...*

One GP had uncertainties about whether symptom control using a syringe driver may shorten a patient's life.

> There is no doubt about it in my mind, that when you put up a syringe driver, very often the patient will not live longer than a few days in quite a lot of cases. I'm sure there must be some patients who are actually aware that the syringe driver is going to end their lives. But there certainly are cases where not only quality of life but probably longevity is improved by the fact that they are able to exist more normally.

Patients may relate increasing the dose of morphine with an attempt to speed up the death or with progression of disease.

> It was awkward every time you were increasing the dose, it was like one of those people where, if you are doubling it, oh, does that mean I am getting worse doctor, you know.

This feeling may account for the reluctance of some doctors to prescribe morphine, and for the non-compliance of some patients who are prescribed the drug.

Controlling breathlessness can also cause distress to patients and doctors:

> I think part of it is this business of the breathing with terminally ill patients... I hate that as a symptom, I dislike that as a symptom, that's why I kept sending her back I think.

The doctor finds this symptom distressing and refers the patient back to hospital.

The patient may present a brave face and deny symptoms.

*She had been struggling on without mentioning too much,*
*according to me anyway, with back pain.*

Patients need explanation, not only the correct prescription. They may wrongly associate control of symptoms with control or cure of the underlying cancer.

Cancer patients get symptoms from diseases other than cancer: this can make it difficult for the doctor to know whether to refer. It can be helpful for the GP to share the care with a specialist. However, some doctors continue to struggle with difficult dilemmas without asking for help. Perhaps they feel a sense of failure, or fear that specialist teams will take over care.

Specialist advice can enable symptoms to be controlled, dispel morphine myths and give the patient an opportunity to express psychological and spiritual concerns. Specialists can support doctors as well as patients when pain is difficult to relieve:

*I spoke to the specialist quite a lot on the phone and she was*
*really helpful.*

## Suffering and hope

The pioneering work of hospices has led to improvements in the care of patients with advanced cancer. However, there are dying patients who suffer distress which is not relieved by medical treatment. Unrelieved suffering presents ethical dilemmas for patients, families, healthcare professionals and society.

Suffering is a subjective concept, which is familiar to each of us, yet is difficult to define. It involves factors which diminish quality of life, a perception of distress and an expression of a life not worth living.[67]

Suffering is a threat to a patient's autonomy. Moreover, suffering is not limited to the patient but extends to involve the family and healthcare professionals. It is not directly related to the severity of symptoms but depends on more subtle factors, such as whether a person has come to terms with dying, the quality of their support and their previous personality. A strong need for control, for instance, may exacerbate a patient's suffering.

Isolation and pain can lead to feelings of low self-esteem and loss of hope. Hopelessness is a state characterised by an inability to anticipate any positive outcome. The patient is unable to make decisions, enjoy meaningful relationships or express joy.[68] Hopelessness is a source of suffering.[24]

Hope may be increased by feeling valued as a person in a meaningful relationship and by setting realistic goals. Several doctors expressed difficulty in achieving a balance between maintaining realistic hopes and being over-optimistic:

> The line I try to take is to hear how they feel about it, I don't want to dampen people's positive outlook on things because I'm sure that can be of benefit but just perhaps to gently introduce the ideas of, are they doing as well as they think?

The GP may become unpopular in trying to lower unrealistic expectations.

> I distinctly remember a lady with an ovarian carcinoma who I wanted to make comfortable but who was clinging to the hope of a cure which never existed. Because of this hope she let herself submit to chemotherapy for quite a long time which was making her quite uncomfortable. Now that conflict made it difficult and eventually she ditched me as her GP.

False hope is the creation of an expectancy that an unlikely outcome is probable. It is sometimes created to soften the emotional impact of a difficult situation. On the other hand, false despair may be a purposeful lowering of the patient's expectations to avoid future disappointment.

Over-optimism may present as unrealistic expectation of cure:

> ...and she was inappropriately optimistic, well I'm going to fight this and I'm sure I'm going to do all right...

False hopes lead to the patient avoiding completing unfinished business or to the persistence of denial:

> I didn't say he was going to be cured but I really wasn't feeling that perhaps it was in his best interest to try and fill him in entirely as to what the prognosis was.

Working with the patient at his own pace and acknowledging his coping strategies is one way of fostering hope. Conflicts can occur when the patient's need for hope differs from those of the professionals.

Many patients are realistic about their future. Cassileth et al. found that patients were able to maintain hope, and in general were more hopeful despite having information about their diagnosis.[69]

> Her expectations were quite realistic really. She had this idea that she would gradually fade away over the next 12 months and that's really what happened.

Some patients seem to give up:

> Undoubtedly it can happen, and I have seen it happen, where people have been so distressed by the fact that they just think, well that's it.

Flemming noted in her study that patients close to death seemed to 'hang on' for particular events such as a birthday or a family anniversary. Conversely, there were patients who gave up and died much sooner than one would have expected.[70] Flemming concluded that the influencing factor in each case was the presence or absence of hope.[70]

Humour may be a way to maintain hope in certain patients.

> *It's almost like flirting with a girl, you partly saying things that are provocative and the other person knows they are not true. Its part of a game and I remember one person, again with lung cancer, where I said well everybody just loves to come visiting you so you are going to have to carry on a bit. That, I knew in a way that there is some truth in that but it was also partly in jest but it wasn't enough reason really to give her to carry on but we just played a game. It was part of a banter between doctor and patient that just shows that even in the midst of this seriousness that you can still play around with words and feelings.*

Patients and relatives may push for aggressive anticancer treatment mainly to maintain hope. Goals of treatment in advanced cancer should be to maintain mobility and continence, relieve pain and suffering, support dignity, and protect the ability to think. Such a policy protects scarce resources and spares patients. Realistic assessment of risk-benefit and cost-benefit ratios in the care of each patient may avoid unnecessary treatments given to maintain hope.

Physicians need to define what treatment is appropriate, not what treatment is possible. When economies are being made, it is common to save on relatively low profile aspects of treatment such as psychosocial support of cancer patients.

In Flemming's study, hope was influenced by the ability of the patient to have a sense of control over the disease and treatment. The most important factor was the presence of medical and nursing staff.[70] In maintaining a desire to continuing living, the support of family and friends is crucial. In the next chapter, their needs are explored.

# CHAPTER SIX

# SUPPORTING THE
# RELATIVES AND CARERS

*I see in the clothes a symbol of continuing life*
*and proof that I still want to be myself.*
*If I must drool, I may as well drool on cashmere.*

**Jean-Dominique Bauby**

Relatives may have great difficulties accepting that further treatments
are futile.

> When he became terminal that took a long time for them all
> to accept, and the sons didn't really accept it until after he
> had died. That was, they kept asking for things to be done,
> you know, isn't there anything else that could be done to get
> rid of it.

Relatives are anxious about what is going to happen to their loved one,
the manner of dying and the sources of support available to them.

> Their anxiety was how is he going to progress, what
> complications might ensue, how is he going to die, will we be
> able to look after him, what will happen, what help will we get?

> It wasn't so much prognosis but her mode of death that he was
> worried about, what would happen, what should he do, who
> should he call and that sort of thing.

One of the commonest difficulties experienced by the GPs was when
the patient and the relatives had differing rates of acceptance of the
situation.

> One of the things I felt difficult was between the husband and
> the wife's attitude to the illness. She was the patient and she
> accepted the diagnosis very quickly, and quickly adapted
> herself to the palliative stage, once the diagnosis was made,
> that was it, she was going to die. Whereas he was very much
> more along the lines of all that can be done must be done and
> the conflict between them was difficult to manage.

Relatives may react by demanding treatments for the patient.

*It was she who was driving her mother's alternative therapy rather than Mrs R herself. And that was sometimes difficult because, if you like, on whose behalf should I be fighting? You certainly didn't want to be divisive between them.*

Finding the right language to explore or challenge the relatives' view may be a problem.

*It's much easier to say what they want you to say but I think you need to approach it and try and bring out the fact that they have got the wrong idea and he isn't going to get better but that's the difficult bit.*

Patients need to be reassured that they will not be abandoned and to trust their GP.

*...more how they view you as a person I think and whether they think you've just given up on them, whether you just don't care, you know he's going to die and there is nothing else you can do...*

*...you think you're doing all the right things and then they question it all the time and suggest something new...*

Relatives may react with fear.

*Their anxiety was shown as aggression but I went on a couple of evenings and I spent some time at the early stages and I'm sure that paid dividends because I felt then it would be much easier to pop in and out once I'd established a rapport with them.*

Or, they may be angry.

> *Her husband was beside himself with rage because the*
> *specialist hadn't made the diagnosis of carcinoma of her*
> *lung.*

Bereavement care is an essential part of palliative care. Relatives often have a need to express gratitude, although the doctor may not feel it is justified:

> *I do sometimes think that some very very nice things are said*
> *to us after people have died and I hope some of them are*
> *deserved but some of them I don't think probably are and you*
> *wonder whether it's just you're supposed to thank the doctor*
> *and thank the nurses.*

> *There is one that I felt was equally disastrous but for other*
> *reasons and I see this woman's husband and, if someone had*
> *actually overheard the conversation he had with me, you'd*
> *think well, the care must have been wonderful, but it wasn't,*
> *it was absolutely dreadful. The whole situation was almost out*
> *of control the whole time, but he comes along and says all*
> *these marvellous things.*

Bereavement problems often present as physical symptoms.

> *He was a man who was very passive and always seemed to*
> *accept her problem with a shrug of the shoulders and I think,*
> *being an Asian, he would have said, it's the will of God. I*
> *don't think he is particularly religious but he always accepted*
> *it, but he tended to be constantly coming to you, and still is,*
> *with physical symptoms which often have little or no basis but*
> *are obviously an expression of his turmoil...*

The final moments are of particular importance to the relative and may leave a lasting impression of the totality of the quality of care.

*I felt upset about that after, having a misunderstanding at the
end, because I felt really that everyone had been doing their
level best without being appreciated by her, but I think that
she was a bit upset that nobody else was there at the time he
actually died.*

A prolonged dying process may impose particular stresses on the
relatives who may wish to see things speeded up.

*I think you worry about criticism of not doing a good job.
But then, I think relatives panic, this is an awkward position.
I think very often relatives panic and want you to speed
things up.*

Relatives may be frightened of their loved one dying at home and
wish to have them admitted to hospital at the end.

*I had a lot of trouble, in her terminal state, persuading her
husband to hang on to her. I don't know whether that was fair
or unfair... I can actually imagine that a marital bed is an
uncomfortable place to find a dead person.*

*Her husband was massively overprotective and had a rather
irritating demeanour of finding it necessary to demonstrate
how caring he was being, for my benefit while I was there, he
used to cluck and fuss around her, fluff her pillows and get her
a drink.*

Two important factors that help bereaved people are their
involvement in the care of the person who died and the belief that
they received good care.[3] Some problems may be the result of
relatives trying to do something:

*...something must be done, you must be doing something. I'm*

*sure that's an over-riding thing in lots of cases whereas if you
sat back and actually looked at the overall picture one would
think well, does one need to do this?*

Dudgeon et al. studied 150 cancer patients who said their biggest
concern was being a burden to their family.[71] Thus, attempts to
address the patient's main concerns therefore require working with
the family as well as the patients.

Relatives often fear the harm of giving honest information to the
patient. They may insist that the doctor must not tell the patient that
cure is no longer possible. 'The news would kill him, doctor.' Thus
collusion is born, and grows to isolate the patient from his family,
doctor and nurses.

Relatives need time to share their fears and distress. Carers may feel
helpless and think that their loved one is suffering. We need to
acknowledge that they are acting from the best of motives, to preserve
their loved one from harm. Relatives need to discover for themselves
the cost of maintaining deception, a distancing from the patient. Finally
they need help and support in sharing the truth with the patient.

Collusion is difficult to manage but is easier to prevent. If doctors
resolved to discuss the diagnosis with the patient and the relatives
together, then collusion would be less likely to occur. Respect for
autonomy demands that the patient should be the first to know what
is happening to his body. Professionals can help by suggesting that
relatives are present at these discussions.

The relatives may insist that 'something must be done'. Relatives are
often unfamiliar with the features of the normal dying process. They
may have fantasies and fears surrounding issues of terminal
dehydration and starvation.

Changes in family structure have created problems for modern families who wish to fulfil their responsibilities of care.[3] Smaller family size, involvement of women in work outside their homes and the complexities arising from divorce have contributed to a decline in home deaths and an increase in institutionalised death.[3] As Fields comments, 'If the trend continues, home deaths will soon become as rare as home births'.[3]

# CHAPTER SEVEN

# PRACTICAL ISSUES

*In nature there's no blemish but the mind;*
*None can be called deform'd but the unkind*

**William Shakespeare**

## Lack of time

GPs identified that there is a problem in giving patients and their families enough time. One response to this difficulty is to delegate the task to nurses.

> *I don't feel I give enough time myself just to sit and talk to someone. I like to find someone they can identify with, whether it's a District Nurse or a Home Care Assistant or somebody, somebody that they feel has just got time to sit that they can talk to.*

It is interesting to note how professionals undervalue the importance of giving patients time.

> *The other thing is, the more I can't do things the more I go. I'm sure that's guilt, I feel the only thing at the end of the day you have to offer is interest.*

> *I was visiting him once or twice a week at this stage and I'd only been a couple of days before and they'd asked me to go back and it was totally inappropriate...*

Howie et al. have looked at factors which empower patients in consultations with their GPs. One of the most significant positive factors was the duration of the consultation.[77] The authors advocate rewarding doctors who spend more time with their patients.

## Continuity of care

The GPs identified a problem in maintaining continuity of care in patients with advanced cancer.

> *Continuity can be a hell of a problem for the doctor sometimes, no doubt about that, not just because there are a*

*lot of people with a lot of visiting required, if you're having to go several times a week to somebody, if you're busy it can be a hell of a business and not only that, also it's a stress emotion isn't it. Sometimes it helps to have more than one person going in. But I think from the patient's point of view and from the relatives, I think they do like continuity of care and I think it's reasonable and right they should have a reasonable degree of continuity of care.*

*I think that terminal care is probably if not the most important then certainly one of the most important things that GPs can become involved in. I do feel very strongly that there should be continuity of care with patients you've known in the past and have been involved in the diagnosis. I feel it's that personal involvement that is often the most important thing, from feedback from the patient and the relatives, that there is one person there, who is very continuously who you can turn to, who you learn to trust, who can really take control of the situation.*

Despite this, out of hours and weekend cover is provided by others.

*I think it is quite a problem when you get to this stage. He was very close to dying and I thought he was going to die before I left and it is difficult. I think they got to know most of the partners throughout the time because of weekends and nights, but I'm sure it is more difficult especially for the family because they get to know you and they were the people having the most problems with it all, and then somebody new comes in that they don't know and they doubt them again, are they doing the right things... I think they'd just started to trust me and to believe what I was saying and then somebody else comes along.*

*Continuity of care has been a problem for me. I feel that whenever I have got somebody who is terminally ill, that I have got a special responsibility and yet despite that I think that there has been a failure in continuity of care. I think there are two reasons for that, one is the way the practice is set up… we tend to take equal numbers of visits. The other factor was a personal factor which was that I was away doing a course plus spending a day out of the practice.*

The involvement of different doctors can lead to problems due to lack of communication and differing prescribing practices.

*Whoever was on call was getting called most evenings and so they were just increasing the MST, so I wasn't completely in control of the dose and it just kept getting put up over weekends and things until he was actually toxic with it.*

With the increasing use of GP co-operatives to cover out of hours work it becomes even more likely that dying patients could see a number of different doctors who are not familiar with their history or care. While this may not be critical in acute illness, continuity of care is an essential ingredient of high quality palliative care.

Doctors may find that, because they cannot do any more active treatment, they make too many home visits.

*You can go in to see them too often, I find that, and then there isn't anything to do and it looks as if you're just calling in all the time and not doing anything. It's difficult to know how often to go and how much to do, isn't it.*

The frequency and rationale for home visiting was a source of stress.

*I feel uneasy about the quality of care when there is more than one visit a day. I suppose then you are reaping the consequences of your failure to sort out his psychological needs.*

*I make my working day for hard for myself doing a lot of this. I think it's probably, I make up in time for what I lack in perhaps, ability or knowledge or dealing with the disease and I try to give them time instead.*

Some patients wish to retain as much control as possible.

*In fact normally, I think we're bloody good on continuity of care and terminal care and I would say, I think the problem is that until a month before she died, she was dictating when she was coming rather than us saying I'll see you in such and such a time. Under those circumstances it's possible she will see different people at different times.*

*In those last weeks I was there nearly every day and even not counting the emotional stress involved in that, it's just the sheer fact that you've got someone to see, you know it's half an hour a day, to have one patient that you've got to see every day for however many weeks.*

## Promoting effective teamwork

Palliative care demands a multidisciplinary team approach, and this can lead to problems, for example, in taking time to plan care which later becomes inappropriate.

*I've found before with palliative care, you'd get an idea about something, try and get it all set up and two months later or whatever, it all becomes completely irrelevant, but whether it helps all of us to be busy arranging things I don't know.*

Sometimes doctors feel that too many professionals are involved.

> *I think it's very easy to get steamed up about things like that and I find it frustrating when there are people who are not doctors involved in their management.*

A balance needs to be found so that there are not too many professionals involved in the care.

> *I think all of us were pretty impressed with the relationship we have with the specialist nurse in terminal care. One of the problems about having a team approach is, I always feel worried having a large number of people involved.*

> *I thought my relationship and the nurses' relationship was quite good and I suppose I saw it as a failure of what we were trying to do if, at the end, she was admitted into hospital for half an hour, because it looked at this stage that he wanted her admitted. I persuaded him it was a good idea to have a Marie Curie nurse to sit in at very short notice and they were brilliant in fact.*

District Nurses have a key role in providing palliative care at home.

> *I think the most important thing is the District Nurses... We have a stethoscope and a white coat and hover about in the background like God somewhat and yet the nurses are actually bearing much more of an emotional brunt than we are, I imagine. I don't know but I think in some ways it's tougher to be a nurse dealing with the dying and the bereaved.*

> *I think our nurses, we all work together very well. I'm always interested to get input from them about their feelings of what is happening. We all tend to work in the same direction and they come to us appropriately. I'm not so sure with the*

> *hospital, I feel it's silly sending them back to the hospital*
> *clinic because they are rushing in and out with lots of people*
> *with curative things.*

Though in any team there is potential for conflict:

> *There is a District Nurse I've worked with that sometimes you*
> *do feel slightly that 'I care more, I visit more', which I suppose*
> *is partly my own paranoia...*

Some GPs felt they had a role in co-ordinating and integrating care.

> *I think, looking back, I could have provided more focusing,*
> *drawing the various strings together in terms of other people*
> *who were involved.*

## The interface between primary and secondary care

Some GPs felt they ought to have had a greater influence in decision-making.

> *I would say it was a disaster really, on reviewing it. I cannot*
> *justify my failure to argue in that respect. What's going on,*
> *what are we going to achieve?*

General practitioners can feel marginalised by hospital colleagues and lose touch with their patients.

> *I'm sure they looked after him nicely in hospital, but I felt I'd*
> *lost touch with him really.*

Fundholding also creates problems.

> *Fundholding is a total dilemma like that, I think, because you*
> *are being forced to think about your population not an*
> *individual.*

*...in the wonderful world of fundholding now you tend to get more quick correspondence with less and less information.*

Communications between hospitals and GPs were cited as inadequate and a source of uncertainty. Hospital letters, in particular, come in for criticism.

*There is always a confusion in hospital letters, you have to read between the lines, they may well have been told that they have got cancer, but you don't know from reading the letter, the degree of detail they have...*

*My criticism of the letters is that they often stick things in sentences that hold more than one idea and it may be that they told the patient something to do with the malignancy but didn't tell them exactly everything.*

The language also comes in for criticism.

*I think it would be much more useful to have something more along the lines of guidelines in prognosis, and just a sentence to say we'll see him any time should his effusion need tapping or something like that.You feel it's always very difficult to get the information you want out of it.The letters always seem to become very sparse I find once they reach a terminal phase. The amount of useful, caring information doesn't seem to be very much.*

Consultants come in for both criticism and praise:

*If you're sharing uncertainties with perceived experts it's very easy really...*

*I think generally, Dr X [a consultant] is somebody who I*

*really respect as being on the good side of directness and at the same time not lacking subtlety as far as consultants go.*

*He is somebody who is not getting full marks for sensitivity but getting very good marks for directness and honesty and integrity, and at the same time as he gives bad news he allows them to have confidence. He is very paternalistic, you know, trust in me, sort of thing, it's not a bad combination.*

Admitting patients to hospital can be difficult and a source of great stress for GPs.

*I rang up the Medical Houseman on call and said could we admit to EMU and he said yes fine, and I got a phone call a few minutes later from the medical consultant saying no you can't.*

The diagnosis was sometimes made in hospital and problems occurred because GPs did not feel they were always informed.

*One of the problems with patients like her who attend the hospital regularly, is that we don't always get a clear record of what happened.*

# CHAPTER EIGHT

# SOURCES OF STRESS
# FOR DOCTORS

*Strange to know nothing, never to be sure*
*Of what is true or right or real*

Philip Larkin

Doctors feel a personal burden of caring and admit to feelings of inadequacy.

> *I'm very mechanistic with terminal care. I'm not very good with emotional things, I'm not a good counsellor.*

> *He chose me as the person with whom he wanted to have this sort of care but it was a bit difficult. I don't think I really did enough.*

They acknowledge the difficulty of this type of work:

> *I think it can be very taxing because often you are having to go back to see patients and relatives very frequently over quite a long period of time. It's physically taxing, it's emotionally taxing, and it's intellectually taxing, knowing what's the best thing to do sometimes.*

Palliative care is not highly technical but it challenges us ethically. Some doctors are uncertain whether they have shortened a patient's life.

> *...whether I did right, I put her on chlorpromazine to try to reduce that distress. Over the next 24 hours she became rapidly terminal.*

Most doctors felt guilty and feared being blamed for any delay in making a diagnosis.

> *She wanted me particularly to call, and my instant paranoid thought was that she was going to complain that I'd missed it, but that wasn't it at all, she just wanted to talk over her worries about what was happening.*

These fears are likely to increase with political pressure to diagnose cancer at the earliest possible stage.

*I think there is increasing pressure all the time, particularly in recent years, to get the diagnosis right early. The patients expect that and their expectations are much higher than five or ten years ago. I find that a great pressure, you wonder what they're thinking . . .*

There was a feeling that patients did not appreciate just how much uncertainty there is in medical practice. Some doctors felt that patient's expectations of them posed a problem.

*Increasing expectation is the stress that I feel. That's a common perception, you're trained so you must know the answer, you're trained to do it, get the answer right or you're somehow below par. The fact that there are so many grey areas and so much uncertainty, I think that people don't appreciate.*

*I often feel acutely aware and frustrated that people expect us to be much better than we actually are. I do have a horrendous need to feel that other people think I'm being helpful.*

Finding out that a patient has cancer is stressful for professionals as well as for patients and their families.

*When she found that she had a lump on her breast, at first I tried to reassure her because it felt like a cyst to me and XX also thought it was, but to everybody's consternation it proved to be a carcinoma.*

*Well, like everybody, [I felt] totally stunned and disbelieving at first, and had long talks about it because I'd known her so well previously.*

Doctors may find it difficult because they want the patient to survive and have feelings of anger and guilt.

> *I felt that I definitely owed him one and I definitely wanted things to go as smoothly as they possibly could and I think that's why I got increasingly upset when things didn't seem to go smoothly.*

It is difficult to find the balance between reassuring the patient and making them aware of the need to return if signs of disease recur. The doctor may feel a sense of blame.

> *I was horrified when she came back with this enormous lump and felt should I have emphasised the need to return more.*

As in the earlier phases of care, doctors had feelings of guilt about their level of care.

> *...it was the guilt initially that had I missed the diagnosis and then this business of being away during the terminal phase. Had I just not recognised how terminal she was, and one of my partners had to do that for me, or whether the situation had changed in my absence.*

Another doctor's story illustrates how much effort some GPs put into providing personalised care at the end of people's lives.

> *I used to try and draw up with them the days that I work and the days that I don't and give them my home phone number and that sort of thing, and explain what they should and shouldn't do and who to contact if I'm not available. I always give them a named doctor for the days that I'm not at work.*

Doctors have different ways of coping with uncertainty.

*I think you have to be able to handle that uncertainty and I think I always have. I've never found the need to tie up all the ends of everything in any part of my life, so I don't think that's been a problem for me in general terms. I just spotlight it as an increasing pressure.*

A GP offers thoughts about how he copes with the uncertainty of decision-making at this time, by acknowledging uncertainty and involving the patient in the care:

*With increasing years in general practice I think I reduce the amount that I flannel or bullshit or try to appear to have more knowledge than I have got really.*

GPs' own attitudes to palliative care affect their care. Age and experience can be of benefit.

*Just a few more years in a job makes you possibly slightly less insecure about lack of knowledge really… there is a background of faith or confidence that faced with an unusual situation, you'll manage it appropriately.*

The level of stress in caring for a dying patient may be revealed by the sense of relief which may occur at the time of the patient's death.

*Whenever these patients do die there is always a sense of relief. You think, thank God, because it does begin to get to you.*

Doctors, like everybody, carry their own losses. It may be difficult at times to support relatives when you are grieving.

*At the time that XX died my father had just died and that all seemed to get tied up for me really. I remember going around to see Mrs XX afterwards and I was fine, I'm usually all right talking about these things, I sometimes find myself*

*brimming a little bit, but I can usually control that and then*
*she said something that got to me and I actually got upset, I*
*couldn't help it. It was really mixed up with my own*
*problems, my own father. Then I felt doubly guilty because she*
*was comforting me...*

However, expressing emotions is no bad thing. We encourage others
to do it, but tend to pretend that professionals are immune to
distress. Fortunately, our patients and their families understand and
appreciate that doctors sometimes cry too.

*I usually manage to keep things very separate. I didn't in that*
*case, but as I said, I don't think it mattered really. People like*
*to think you're involved and have a great opinion of their*
*husband or father, you don't always need to hide your*
*emotions.*

Age has its compensations.

*That's one of the advantages of being an old GP, you tend to*
*handle situations better and you've got a more authoritative*
*manner. I've found that true in all sort of areas of the*
*practice, that's about the only benefit I can think of for*
*getting old.*

Acknowledging uncertainty is essential, but it may unsettle some
patients.

*I think sometimes I frighten people by seeming uncertain*
*when actually they want you to be quite assertive in a way.*
*I've sometimes thought that people have thought, oh she*
*doesn't know what she's doing, and it's when you've been*
*more open in your uncertainties than in fact was appropriate.*

Talking and listening to patients is a vital part of the doctor's job. Yet some GPs feel guilty for spending time.

> *I do worry. I sometimes think the only good I do in this room is talking to people, but then I do sometimes think, well hang on a minute, you are actually supposed to do a job as well...*

Although doctors work in partnerships, palliative care can be isolating.

> *...general practice is terribly isolated like that, just trying to make a decision on your own and seeing where they've not worked...*

Others are able to share with their colleagues:

> *I think I'm reasonably clear – I never feel lonely in these situations.*

> *I don't feel nurses are very helpful but probably only a GP sees it from a GP point of view.*

Doctors may find it helpful to share their suffering with a colleague.

> *I've got a young woman at the moment who is only 39 with a carcinoma of the lung who has developed an obstruction despite all sorts of treatment. I can see that she is not going to die very quickly, her symptoms are distressing. Yes, I think it is stressful, I think it's one of the major stresses really when you are doing your best and someone is in pain and distress and you don't seem to be able to adequately relieve it. I find it very useful to talk to my colleagues about this, we all tend to chat about it, about what we can do. It's quite useful to share ideas about it. I think perhaps I should sometimes look for*

more help, more expert advice. You tend to get bogged down with a patient. You're looking after them yourself, you are going continuously yourself, going on and on and on seeing them, you tend to lose the thread of what's going on. Sometimes it helps for someone else to come in, say one of your partners. It's not just with this but all sorts of care, a lot of us get so involved in things we forget what we are aiming for sometimes.

# CHAPTER NINE

# FRAMEWORKS OF
# DECISION-MAKING

*Life is short, science is long;*
*Opportunity is elusive, experience is dangerous,*
*judgement is difficult*

**Hippocrates**

Rapid advances in cancer treatments and the search for cures have created a division between scientific technical care, which is based on evidence from populations, and personalised palliative care, which looks at the individual and his family. These differing approaches have evolved their own philosophies of care, resulting in tensions between objective curative treatment and empathetic palliative care, between concepts of curing and caring.

This study of general practitioners reveals many dilemmas for patients, relatives and professionals. We need a better understanding of the process of decision-making in order to develop a framework to help professionals to improve care.

A framework functions as an intellectual device that simplifies and clarifies the source of uncertainty and suggests an ethical approach to decision-making. We need to develop a model which combines scientific competence with respect for the patient's autonomy and compassion – a framework of practical wisdom.

It is helpful to begin by examining some existing frameworks of medical decision-making.

## Ethical frameworks

### Utilitarianism and deontology

Ethical frameworks based purely on abstract theories of deontology or utilitarianism may seem hard to apply in an individual clinical context. Utilitarianism, which advocates the greatest good for the majority, seems to discriminate against the individual cancer patient. On the other hand, the impersonal duties of deontological theory may not be appropriate for the emotional aspects of the care of a patient who is suffering. Both these theories place great emphasis on pure reasoning and seem to reject and mistrust emotions. They also seem to ignore the practical effects of the difference in power between professionals and their patients.

## Autonomy, beneficence, non-maleficence and justice

Similarly, models based on the quartet of autonomy, beneficence, non-maleficence and justice are useful in abstract analysis but less helpful at the bedside where they often conflict. The clinician is still faced with making a value judgement as to which duty has precedence in resolving a dilemma.[61,72]

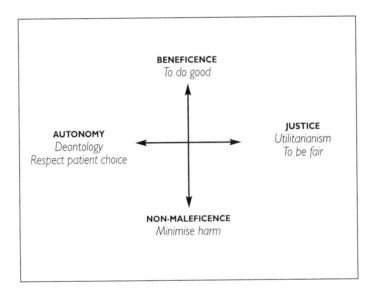

## Respect for autonomy

George et al. have devised a model of decision-making based on respect for patient autonomy.[6] Respecting autonomy means that patients share a responsibility for the decisions they make with their professional advisors. This framework stresses the importance of a good quality of life for the individual.

George's model involves a visual way of applying a therapeutic index, balancing cost against benefit as a beam, balancing curative (pathology based) and palliative (symptom based) options on a fulcrum (patient's agenda).

| CURATIVE<br>(Pathology Based) | PATIENT AGENDA | PALLIATIVE<br>(Symptom Based) |
|---|---|---|
| DIAGNOSIS | TASKS | WASTED TIME |
| CURABILITY | RELATIONSHIPS | SIDE EFFECTS |
| PROGNOSIS | UNFINISHED BUSINESS | COMPLICATIONS |
| BUYING TIME | POLYPHARMACY | BUYING QUALITY |

George et al. suggest that clinical decision-making is more difficult when it is certain that the patient will die despite our best efforts.[6] However, this study shows that great uncertainty exists at all stages of disease, when clinicians may be caught in a dilemma between over-treating patients on the one hand, or neglecting some remote chance of cure on the other. There is a need to balance buying time with buying quality of life.

The legitimacy of buying time may be reasonable. There is a need to explain the costs of going down the curative side, in terms of unfinished business, tasks, relationships and personal resolution. Because the boundaries of care are blurred, it may be more appropriate to shift our attention to respect for the patient's autonomy.

# Mechanistic and probabilistic models of Bursztajn et al[72]

### The mechanistic model

This framework is based on the Newtonian scientific paradigm: cause and effect relationships can be known with certainty. This kind of thinking is grounded in the belief that given a particular cause for distress, a particular procedure will bring relief, e.g. large bowel obstruction will be relieved by a colostomy. Mechanistic approaches search for one causative factor, and carry out tests to isolate and measure one cause at a time. Treatment can only start with a definite diagnosis. In reality, however, treatment can be part of the diagnostic process. The mechanistic clinician does not allow his beliefs, attitudes and values to affect his practice.

When one's thinking is guided by the mechanistic model, with its unattainable standard of certainty, one becomes anxious when one has to take chances. The option of facing uncertainty may be less attractive than the illusion of certainty and control offered by the mechanistic model. It is difficult for people to think rationally when they are scared. This applies as much to a patient receiving bad news as to a doctor facing a difficult prognostic question. In this situation there is a risk that both patient and doctor may become more rigid in their thinking. There are several decision-making models which rely on mechanistic thinking.

### Theoretical decision analysis

This provides ways of setting out a sequence of choices and their possible outcomes.[73] It involves presumptions that have their origin in the mechanistic paradigm. It can be both an aid and a barrier to critical thinking. If it takes into account chance, choice, probability and value then by going through the steps of decision analysis doctors become aware of how much these variables affect decisions.

This type of framework does not really clarify situations where there is no single right solution for every patient. The decision trees developed to help management of appendicitis or a fractured femur are not readily transferable to the arena of palliative care because at each step large questions of judgement and individual values arise for both the doctor and the patient. Doctors need to take into account the effects of their own actions as not only observers but participants in the decision. The manner of the doctor can influence the decision the patient makes.

### Algorithms

An algorithm is a sequence of instructions for solving a problem. It may result from repeated decision analyses of similar cases which can then be combined to form strategies. An algorithm may take the form of a general decision tree which can be adapted for the individual patient, thus saving the doctor and patient the time needed to construct a decision tree for each case. However, decision analysis assumes that a series of decisions extending into the future can be structured and anticipated in advance. It is not easy to modify a decision tree when patients change their minds having experienced the consequences of earlier decisions. In real life, as this study shows, decisions are influenced by unexpected events, professional conflicts, poor communications, lack of time and resources and family problems.

Decision analyses are limited by the data quality of data. Data always carries some degree of uncertainty. The degree of confidence that one can place in decision analysis depends on the degree of confidence one has in human judgements which are not made more certain by being expressed in numbers. Just as the drunken man in the dark looks for his lost car keys in the lit doorway, rather than where he dropped them, because 'that's where the light is', so the decision analyst may look where their method shines the light rather than where the light needs to be shed.[72]

Decision analysis and algorithms may be of help as a tool to explore options rather than as a way of making a definite choice. Decisions need to involve the patient and family. There is a temptation to use decision analysis in a mechanistic way rather than in a creative manner. Decision trees are unrepresentative of the illogical and inconsistent ways in which people reach a decision.

### Therapeutic risk-benefit ratio

In Ashby's framework model the doctor's role is to evaluate investigation and treatment in terms of the therapeutic ratio of risk/benefit to the patient.[1] It is appropriate to shift the balance of decision-making in the direction of the patient and to balance strategies around their agenda.[6]

Ashby's therapeutic ratio examines the balance between active and palliative care and the cut off points we apply.[1] The concept of risk benefit is established in oncology and relates toxicity, morbidity or mortality to benefit.

Ashby's model assumes that the boundaries between the phases of cancer care are clear and the focus of change is the progression of disease pathology. However this mechanistic view takes little account of the blurring between the boundaries which occurs in reality.[1]

### The probabilistic framework[72]

This model of decision-making enables people to acknowledge their values and the uncertainties inherent in the situation and then to gamble consciously according to scientific principles.

The probabilistic model accepts a degree of uncertainty as an inherent part of reality. It treats facts in terms of people's values. We may be afraid of uncertainty and react by either blocking it out or by seeking reassurance from further treatments. The practical consequences of this are either overtreatment or overinvestigation. We cannot make wise decisions when we deny the existence of uncertainty.

The probabilistic model acknowledges that we change what we look at by the very act of observing it. There exists a continuum of the subjective and objective knowledge. The doctor's knowledge is relevant but so are the patient's knowledge and feelings.

The probabilistic model may reduce costs, as patients become not consumers but partners in care. It may also reduce patient-doctor conflict since the fact that things may go wrong and that it may not be anybody's fault are acknowledged from the outset. Expectations of both parties are thus more realistic since patients and their families are involved in decision-making. Such involvement means that the professionals gain the benefit of the patient's knowledge and support that comes from sharing the therapeutic dilemmas which previously the doctor had borne alone.

It is possible that one of the contrasts between decision-making at the boundaries of palliative care is between mechanistic decision-making in the curative phase and an increasingly probabilistic way of reaching decisions in palliative and terminal care.

Having looked at the different approaches to medical decision-making and with the insights gained from the general practitioners' tales we can now evolve a new model of decision-making in palliative care.

# CHAPTER TEN

# PARTNERSHIPS IN
# PALLIATIVE CARE

## A model for decision-making

*Tread softly, for you tread upon my dreams*

**W B Yeats**

## The journey

The general practitioners' tales have revealed uncertainties at all stages of the patient's journey. The timing of the changes from curative to palliative, and from palliative to terminal approaches to caring, involve complex clinical and moral dilemmas. Principles of decision-making are needed which can be used in the clinical context.

Just as we have seen that the boundaries between the phases of care are not fixed but blurred, so too treatment strategies can overlap. The development of joint working between oncology and palliative care teams would facilitate shared decision-making. The failure of chemotherapy, or radiotherapy, or surgery to cure advanced cancer may cause palliative care physicians to neglect their use when they may be helpful. Conversely, oncologists may feel palliative care is easing a patient into an earlier death than is necessary. A state of two solitudes should not exist. Instead, the two should consult and work together more closely.[74]

There is a need to integrate palliative care at an earlier stage in the disease trajectory. Furthermore, this study shows that general practitioners are uneasy about many aspects of the care they are providing for patients with incurable cancer at home.[75]

Doctors and nurses need to face the moral challenge of sharing access to the patient. One of the factors that distinguishes medical oncologists from palliative care physicians is that the former often have the goal of worthwhile remissions.[26] Care should not be directed towards maintaining interprofessional boundaries but rather to respecting the autonomy of the patient. Sharing information within a team is a means of sharing power and of respecting the autonomy of one's colleagues. Much of palliative care is nursing care and we should protect and preserve this vital caring element of our work. Medically defined interventions, made without input from patients or nursing colleagues, risk neglecting the social, spiritual or psychological needs of the dying patient and tend to focus on disease pathology.

## Patients' decisions

In examining the process of decision-making, one of the first questions to answer is, who should make the decision? This study reveals that some general practitioners felt that decisions to switch from curative to palliative care should be taken by hospital consultants. On the other hand, GPs also complained that they felt left out of decision-making once the patient attended hospital. GPs have a privileged perspective of the patient in the context of their family. A process needs to exist whereby hospital consultants can access this valuable source of information to inform their decisions. GPs felt that patients wanted information and to be involved in decisions about their care, but were sometimes happy to leave the technical decisions to the doctor once they had been fully informed. It seems that any framework for decision-making needs to be flexible enough to accommodate the individual preferences of both the patient and the doctor.

A partnership between the patient and the doctor means that the two parties are working towards a common goal.[76] The relationship should be based on trust, and acknowledge that patients are experts on many aspects of their lives. Doctors may be tempted to act in a paternalistic way to do what they think is best for a vulnerable patient. Paternalism, however, creates dependency.[76] Doctors, while experts in the areas of diagnosis and treatment options, do not have sufficient expertise in the patient's social, psychological or spiritual attitudes, beliefs and values to be able to make choices for them.

Some patients may not want an active role in decision-making because they do not want the responsibility for making the 'wrong' choice. The same patient may express different choices to different doctors, or vary his choice from time to time. The doctor needs to acknowledge this uncertainty by trying to find out when patients want an active role and when they prefer to be more passive. The key is to give patients time and as much information as they need, and never to assume anything. Howie et al. have shown an association between patient enablement and length of consultation and continuity of care.[77]

There was a strong feeling amongst GPs that patients had unrealistic expectations of cure. These expectations could be nurtured merely by continuing to refer patients back to hospital clinics or continuing to give them chemotherapy, even though the professionals know that this is intended for palliative treatment rather than cure.

The needs of the patient are paramount, but the views of relatives should be listened to. Where there is a conflict between these views time needs to be spent exploring the reasons for the differences and giving people time to adjust to new situations.

For doctors and patients to face uncertainty together there has to be trust between them. A framework needs to enable patients to make their own decisions by considering their own probabilities, values and categories for making a decision. The patient, relatives and professionals need to weigh the costs of the treatment against the realistic benefits.

This process can take time and the patient needs to reflect on his choices. It can be frustrating for a professional to have to wait for the patient to make a decision. Doctors need to alter attitudes so that they view watching and waiting and being with the patient as 'doing something'.[78] Continuity of care may be difficult to achieve but GPs are in a unique position to continue visiting patients with advanced cancer. Communication skills and commitment should be valued as highly as diagnostic and treatment skills.

Much decision-making is largely mechanistic and is based on a premise that there is a right answer and a scientific solution to all problems. A better way of coping is by using sophisticated decision-making skills which involve:[72]

- acknowledging the uncertainty
- assessing causes and effects probabilistically
- estimating probabilities and values
- understanding the effect of time
- appreciating the importance of the context on decisions
- dealing with emotions that arise in the course of decision-making
- encouraging the patient and relatives to be partners in decision-making.

One way of applying this model is to seek the patient's informed consent.

## Informed consent

An informed choice can give a patient a sense of being in control. A habit of making choices consciously and recognising a degree of uncertainty in one's choices enhances patient autonomy. The satisfaction derived from exercising one's own autonomy may be more important than making the choice with the highest expected value. Patients do not necessarily make conservative decisions when fully informed about the risks and benefits of treatment options.

Autonomy is a central component of a life worth living. This is best protected by a requirement for informed consent. This model of consent should acknowledge that informed consent, like breaking bad news, is a process by which the patient and the professional come to a clearer understanding of the true situation for a particular patient. Such honest conversations take time.[22]

It may be time to reward doctors who have longer consultations, provide greater continuity of care and both enable more patients and enable patients more.[77]

Moody has argued that formal mechanisms of informed consent may be inadequate for protecting a patient's autonomy.[79] He makes a plea for a concept which he calls negotiated consent, which involves shared decision-making between patient, family and professionals.[79]

Towle modifies this by extending the concept beyond consent to informed shared decision-making.[80] This involves sharing the decision between patient and doctor and ensuring that the best evidence is considered, not only about risks and benefits of treatment options but also about the patient's attitudes and values.[80]

Involving patients in decisions about their treatment or care improves health outcomes.[80,81,82]

The majority of patients with advanced cancer are in an anxious state when they see doctors. In such an anxiety state both comprehension and recall skills are diminished. Open honest communication between staff and patients requires a relaxed atmosphere. In this setting, the mutual respect, trust and friendliness between doctors and nurses can lead to their skills being used in an optimal way.[83] An important role for the doctor is to create an environment where patients can feel comfortable in asking questions and participating in the decision process.

Clinicians need to ascertain the patient's understanding of their disease, their view of the future, their coping strategies and their needs for further information. Healthcare professionals need to know the family context and what role the family has in the patient's decision-making process. If decisions are postponed, the patient and family may be deprived of a chance to confront death and dying together and to use the remaining time in the way in which they wish. Furthermore, it may lead to abnormal grieving in the relatives.

Patients need an explanation of their illness and to be aware of the goals of their treatment. They should be given the opportunity to acknowledge which mode of treatment they are in. Ethical issues are better addressed when treatment protocols contain clear patient-family information packages, clear guidelines on obtaining informed and understood consent, and clear emphasis on quality of life criteria including an assessment of the patient's own life goals. Techniques have been described for quantifying patients' goals and acceptance of risk at varying levels of likelihood of treatment success. Slevin has shown that oncologists vary enormously in their choice of treatment for advanced cancers.[32]

Mackillop also shows that while the patient, doctor and family may share a common understanding initially, as time passes and the cancer progresses patients and physicians may develop divergent views on the aims of the therapy. Patients in a palliative setting who are receiving treatment directed at relieving symptoms may well believe that therapy is aimed at disease control. GPs in this study believed that many patients were not clear about the true aims of treatment.

In making an appropriate transition between a curative and a palliative approach to care, with the patient's consent and comprehension, we need to face issues of death and dying. The attitude of the healthcare professional is a key factor in determining whether patient is informed and what choice the patient makes.

A patient-oriented approach concentrates on the need for full information and sets limits on the doctor's perception and beliefs. In his willingness to inform, a doctor reveals his respect for the patient's autonomy. The central function of informed consent is to ensure a sharing of power and knowledge between doctor and patient. Through this sharing process, patients receive appropriate care from doctors they trust, and doctors gain a deeper understanding of the patient's needs. Informed consent can be viewed as an expression of two elements of care: responsiveness to the patient's wishes and protection from harmful intervention.[84] Informed consent is a dialogue between a patient and a doctor in which both become aware of potential harms and benefits for the patient. Informed consent is thus much more than a granting of permission and involves legal, moral and communication issues.

## Communication

These situations highlight the importance of developing the art of communicating in ways that help patients live with uncertainty.[85]

Physicians may need better communication skills to listen to patient preferences and to respond to their needs at the end of life.[68] Medical interventions may fail because many determinants of the doctor's behaviour are more influential than patient preferences. Decisions may be driven by beliefs about treatment efficacy, perceived standards of care, tumour response or prognostic uncertainty.

A continuum exists from advocacy and empowerment, through persuasion, to making the decision for others.[79] The context of the communication between patient, family and professional is an ethical issue. The parties involved must have honest information and an opportunity to negotiate and reflect on their choices. This model recognises that the real world is filled with uncertainty and conflicting interests.[79]

The affect of the doctor and the manner of the communication are crucial in influencing patient's choices. If the doctor feels a sense of failure, and that palliative care equates with giving up, then the patient rapidly picks this up from non-verbal cues. Delegation of this vital explanation and discussion to nurses may be the only pragmatic way of giving patients information, but doctors must have checked that the nurses have the knowledge to answer the therapeutic questions which arise, and offer follow-up support to their nursing colleagues. Good communication skills include listening to the patient, avoiding distancing, sharing emotional involvement and compassion with the patient and family.

There is a need to improve communication skills of healthcare professionals.

It is possible that many individuals would be able to die at home, with their families, without the use of expensive technology if they were well informed and allowed to choose the place in which they are going to die.

Predicting when death is going to occur was a difficulty experienced by many GPs. This uncertainty makes it difficult to resist the application of aggressive treatments which have little chance of success rather than confronting the difficult emotional area of helping patients and their relatives to come to terms with the reality of their situation. This requires sophisticated communication skills and time.

Patients have uncertainties and often morbid fears about the process of dying. Doctors and nurses need to give patients the opportunity to discuss their specific fears.

Doctors also have their own fears of death and dying. The treatment of cancer may have ceased, but care of the patient carries on until the moment of death. Society needs to reach an agreement on the proper care of the dying and to set standards of appropriate palliative care. Professionals need to improve prognostic skills to time the initiation of palliative care to meet the patient's needs.

## When to stop chemotherapy

We need to recognise the complex trade-offs which have to be made between conflicting aims and the uncertainties which are acknowledged in probabilistic decision-making. The mechanistic model sees disease as a physical disturbance that may be corrected by drugs, radiotherapy or surgery. It sees the patient as a condition rather than as a person. Physician fallibility is apparent when working with patients with advanced cancer. For example, in some patients the more we do in an attempt to restore health the more suffering we cause them. Part of the clinician's skill lies in judging when to withhold aggressive treatment for the benefit of the patient and justifying this decision in the face of pressure from patients, relatives, or colleagues. These pressures are based on unrealistic hope rather than reality.

Saying 'no' is difficult. It is simpler to give way to these pressures and give futile active treatment rather than acknowledging the difficult situation and sharing this with the patient and family. Treatment that fails to produce a benefit irrespective of whether it has an effect is futile.[86] In judging futility, the doctor discusses with the patient and family the effect of treatment, which is limited to part of the body, and benefit, which improves the patient as a whole. Doctors are not legally or morally obliged to offer futile treatments.

Giving chemotherapy as a way of maintaining hope or because a patient or relative demands it does not seem to be an ethical use of scarce resources. Time spent with patients and relatives setting realistic goals should be seen as worthwhile work for doctors.

These discussions and those involving the cessation of active treatment require sensitive communication skills and great compassion from the doctors and nurses. If there is insufficient time, or if doctors lack these, skills then there is a danger that advancing cancer is perceived solely as a biological problem requiring even more aggressive drug therapy. Clinical trials of chemotherapy tend to measure success in terms of a reduction in mortality. However, we now need to develop more subtle outcome measures which can reflect gains in the patient's quality of life. Such gains should involve more than a mere reduction in the side effects of chemotherapy.

There are clear protocols for curative treatments in choriocarcinoma, non-Hodgkins lymphoma, Hodgkins disease, germ cell tumours and childhood malignancies. Most adult patients with solid tumours, however, are treated with palliative chemotherapy which aims to improve quality of life. There is still no consensus for best practice in this large group of patients, particularly when the disease is advanced.

Despite poor response rates for metastatic solid tumours, cytotoxic drugs are often used in clinical settings in which there is only meagre evidence of quality of life benefit. Little is known about the quality of life of patients having chemotherapy compared with 'best supportive care', a concept which itself has not yet been defined or generally accepted. Even in patients who do receive symptom control of malignancy, we do not know which cancer-related symptoms are alleviated by chemotherapy and which are not. It may be that skilled support rather than cytotoxics would be more appropriate for some patients and families faced with the realisation that the cancer is now beyond cure.

Where therapies become increasingly aggressive, the patient may die as a consequence of treatment, for example with neutropenic sepsis. In medicine, unlike other aspects of life, doctors are considered much less culpable for killing than for failing to save a life. This may be one factor which drives some doctors to suggest chemotherapy even when the patient is dying. Doctors have a strong sense of their duty of beneficence and this can sometimes translate into paternalistic actions taken for the patient's own good and without their full informed consent, such as pursuing active treatments when the cancer is advanced.

On the other hand some patients may plead for further active treatments. Slevin's study indicates that patients will clutch at straws. We need to identify the group of patients with metastatic cancer who receive little or no benefit from chemotherapy compared with best palliative care. Endpoints in chemotherapy trials often relate to antitumour activity or mortality, with no evidence of the impact of treatment on the patient's quality of life. Moreover, quality of life measures do not adequately reflect the patient's true situation.

It is hard to decide when to switch to palliative care.[17] It may be hard to acknowledge that we cannot do any more and professionals may have feelings of anxiety and guilt. Decisions need to be considered in the context of the individual clinical case and not only in abstract isolation. It is the doctor rather that the nurse who makes the decision to change from a curative to a palliative approach.

Resources in cancer care have been mainly spent on the early phases of prevention, diagnosis, and curative treatments. However, the majority of cancer patients will go on to die of their disease, some in pain, without dignity, and as a burden to their family.

Patients, doctors and nurses often express concern about the value of cytotoxics in incurable cancer. They also question how appropriate it is to investigate patients with end stage disease. The costs to patients of physical toxicity, psychological morbidity, social disruption and economic loss need to be weighed against the benefits of likely tumour regression, symptom relief, improved activity, and prolongation of life.

Published trials may need to be supplemented by scrutiny of the collective experience of clinicians.[87,89]

The intention of palliative chemotherapy is morally relevant to this debate. To justify using palliative chemotherapy, one or more of following criteria should exist:

- *Relief of symptoms* – if the patient has no symptoms then the use of chemotherapy is questionable
- *Prevention of problems* – pulmonary metastases and prevention of breathlessness
- *Prolongation of good quality life not prolongation of suffering* – not often achieved with palliative chemotherapy with the exceptions of small cell lung cancer and ovarian cancer.

## Relief of suffering

Suffering may be seen as a problem to manage, and the process of dying may then become a progression of problems to confront.[2] There is a risk that this distances us from the immediacy of the patient's experience. Medical language reflects our attitudes and reinforces remoteness and distance. Financial pressures and constraints of time work against the humanisation of medical care. Doctors and nurses are universally perceived to be busy. Doctors have their own fears of death and dying and these may lead them to distance themselves from dying patients in order to retain control of their own feelings.[26]

Distancing may take the form of not making time available and keeping the conversation limited to enquiries about symptoms. There is also a risk that patient care of a non-technical nature could be delegated to the least trained. Thus there may be less care available for a suffering patient today, while at the same time technological advances may prolong the dying process.

There have been a number of cases recently in which patients who only wanted standard palliative care have felt it necessary to go to court to be assured of receiving it.[89] The prospect of an undignified, prolonged, painful dying that has generated fear in the minds of patients and has rekindled interest in the possibility of legalising euthanasia.

Similar, uncertainty surrounds the distinction between the administration of sufficient medication to treat suffering and taking part in euthanasia. Such uncertainty results in inadequate control of distressing symptoms and may contribute to the public's increasing demand for legal euthanasia. Addressing attitudinal influences on the care of dying patients requires fundamental shifts in the life-prolonging ethos of medicine.

If we are to improve this situation there is a need to:

- educate doctors and the public about the legitimacy of prescribing analgesia and withdrawing life-sustaining treatments and the distinction between these decisions and euthanasia[90]
- establish standards for futile care
- educate the public on the limitations of medical technology and on the notion of a peaceful death
- improve communication skills in the context of terminal illness when the achievement of a peaceful death assumes priority over prolongation of life.

To restore a balance between a doctor's obligation to prolong life and his obligation to relieve suffering, a peaceful death must be acknowledged as a legitimate goal of medicine. With increased public awareness has come a demand for new standards of end of life care that are better tailored to meet the needs of dying patients. For instance, patients with written Do Not Resuscitate orders continue to receive many other types of medical treatment which have no effect on quality of life.

Two broad approaches have developed to meet the dilemma of intractable suffering. There are those who support the legalisation of active euthanasia and others advocating the development of palliative care. Both the pro-euthanasia lobby and those opposed to the adoption of euthanasia have at the root of their argument a desire to relieve suffering.

A doctor who attempts to kill a suffering patient intends active euthanasia. The arguments surrounding the adoption of active euthanasia for those patients whose suffering is unrelieved is beyond the scope of this study.

The goals and principles of palliative care are logically incompatible with euthanasia. As Farsides points out, we need to be aware that respect for autonomy may have limits if the patient requests euthanasia.[91] Other ethical values take on greater significance in this situation.[92] The trust between both doctors and patients is under threat in many spheres of medicine, as demonstrated by the increasing numbers of cases of litigation and complaints against doctors.

Why is it that many patients no longer trust their doctors? Perhaps the explicit market forces that have been brought into healthcare have contributed to the patients' sense of uncertainty. Some patients are now suspicious that doctors are not acting solely in their best interests and are concerned that clinical decisions are being taken on purely financial grounds.

An ethical response acknowledges the value of the individual's life and the complexity of the concept of suffering. Suffering may not be relieved in the sense that doctors can alleviate all distress, but an ethical response can be made.

## Care

Caring involves the capacity to feel for another person and requires not only an openness to the patient's needs but also a readiness to reflect on the way professionals make judgements about what is best for the patient. Care should be supportive rather than intrusive.

Recognition of a natural dying process is central to the ethics and practice of palliative care. The focus of control of suffering is with the patient, not with professionals. Suffering is an experience which may be helped by others who can provide conditions that assist a patient to come to terms with their suffering, but they cannot control another's suffering. Understanding, empathy and compassion are ethical alternatives to control. Careful assessment requires time along with education in clinical assessment skills and in communication.

Only a minority of patients who need specialist palliative care have access to these services. We need to make the public, politicians and our colleagues aware of what can be achieved by palliative care. If we are truly concerned about the quality of dying then palliative care services need appropriate resources.

## Compassion

In palliative care the doctor patient relationship is a therapeutic tool, and emotion and conflict often arise. Doctors need to learn not to separate the emotional aspects from the clinical but to acknowledge uncertainty.

To 'suffer with' is the root meaning of the word 'compassion'. Suffering enforces isolation: people are severed from familial and social relationships. The presence of a doctor or nurse represents an opportunity to share the vulnerability and suffering of another. Healthcare professionals need time to discover the inner resources available to the patient and to evaluate the patient's coping mechanisms. Time is needed to follow up and to listen carefully to the patient's view. Such time spent needs to be valued by the purchasers and providers of care as much as it is by patients.

This may be uncomfortable for the doctor who needs to acknowledge uncertainty and vulnerability. There is a place here for practical wisdom rather than algorithms to aid decision-making. Imagination may be a potent tool for the clinician.[2] Receptive imagination is a way of achieving empathy, to look at the world from behind the eyes of the patient, and requires a willingness to share the pain: 'I can only imagine what you are going through'.

Doctors need the chance to discuss difficult issues with their colleagues. The emotions, values and intuitions of the doctor endorse the sanctity and value of life. Once judgements about the value of another's life are made, euthanasia becomes a possibility.

## Committment

Patient involvement is crucial if we are to reduce the sense of helplessness and to enhance the feeling of control. The treatment of the cancer may have ceased, but the care of the patient continues until the moment of death. The goal is to make life more meaningful and satisfactory, even if the steps appear to be very small in our eyes. In the patient's eyes these steps matter greatly. We need to be clear as to whose suffering is it we are wanting to treat: is it the patient's, the family's or our own?[94] For doctors, the sanctity of life doctrine, derived from Judaeo-Christian ethics and the Hippocratic ethos, prohibits killing. Doctors have special duties of beneficence and non-maleficence and to kill a patient is to neglect these duties.[95]

A patient who requests euthanasia may be motivated to do so by a belief that they are a burden to their family.[96] Sometimes this belief may be articulated in terms of unrelieved pain. The existence of a prohibition of euthanasia gives the doctor an opportunity to address these important concerns. 'I acknowledge that you feel you want to die, but that is something I cannot do anything about. Let's look at the issues I might be able to help you with.' The feelings of low self worth, helplessness and hopelessness can now be addressed and often the 'pain' is alleviated.

When suffering persists, our continued commitment necessitates acting without certainty. If one's commitment is subordinated to some allegiance to a detached professional demeanour some suffering will remain untouched.[2] We need to appreciate that doubt is not to be feared but welcomed; as Feynman says, 'doubt is not a blemish upon our ability to know but the essence of knowing'.[93]

It is important to be clear that terminal care has nothing in common with euthanasia, which implies the deliberate intention of ending a life. In the terminal phase of care futile medical treatments should be avoided. All interventions are weighed in terms of their benefit to the patient. However, to refer to this refraining from active treatment in a futile situation as euthanasia is illogical. Worse, it may lead doctors to feel they cannot ask for assistance, thus blocking access to appropriate terminal care. Within the terminal phase doctors operate with a therapeutic ratio that balances symptom relief against a risk of death. Death as a relief may be a truth, but to see it as a treatment modality or as a means of achieving relief is not good terminal care, but euthanasia.[6] We have duties of care to ease suffering but not to hasten or prolong the process of dying.

I believe that we should maintain a barrier against euthanasia and allow no erosion of this rule.[97] There is a moral difference between carrying out euthanasia and withdrawing or withholding futile measures at the end of life. The broad prohibition of euthanasia may seem to preclude moral change in future, but it is because the debate is being linked to one of rationing of resources that it is imperative to draw a line beyond which doctors will not go.

The existence of a prohibition of euthanasia has many advantages for patients. For the patient with cancer, and their family, the world may be perceived as an uncertain and frightening place. They need doctors and nurses whom they can trust to work with them to ensure the best possible quality of life, who acknowledge that much suffering is unrelievable but will still give both competent and compassionate care. In this process, there is acknowledgement of the infinite value of the life of the one who suffers, and an inspiration to the many who care to improve both the standards of palliative care and widen its accessibility.

## A partnership of care

If healthcare professionals work together with the patient in a true partnership of care, respecting his autonomy and seeking his informed and understood consent, then we shall have a better chance of achieving our therapeutic aims, whether they are curative or palliative.

The research reveals difficulties in professional relationships which can raise fears among general practitioners that specialists may take over the care of patients.[98] Hospital care on the other hand may not create a suitable environment for the process of dying.[99] Hospitals have traditionally focussed on treating episodic acute illness and prolonging life; over 50% of patients die in hospitals. Data suggest that hospitals and physicians are not equipped or trained to handle the medical and psychosocial problems that face those who are dying.[90]

For doctors and patients to face uncertainty together there has to be trust between them. We cannot make wise decisions when we deny the existence of uncertainty.

Patients need time for doctors and nurses to listen to their views. Patients want to be able to discuss their treatment choices with doctors. This is not to say that they want sole responsibility for the decision. They may wish to leave it to the doctor to advise on the course of treatment but they want the information so that they may be actively involved in the decision.

## Acknowledge uncertainty

Doctors need to acknowledge that the world changes and the relationship between the world and the decision maker changes. Time and the feelings of the people involved create a fluid context in which decisions are made. As time passes, probabilities, values, feelings and information all may change. The results of one decision affect the next decision. The probabilistic paradigm is one where data must be interpreted by the doctor and patient rather than dictating conclusions. A dilemma would not be a dilemma if the 'best' decision always led to the 'best' outcome. Sometimes a wise strategy does not have a satisfactory outcome.[72] By taking responsibility for one's choices and their consequences one trains oneself to make further choices. Trust fosters this process of decision-making. Trust allows doctor and patient to persist with a decision long enough to assess its long term as well as immediate outcomes; it also gives them time to change their minds. Trust is gained by being with patients, acknowledging uncertainty and vulnerability and by being available to patients.

One of the most important advantages of working within a team is that the decision may be discussed with other team members.[100] There is no such thing as unbiased, impartial information in medicine. Is the glass half full or half empty? If the doctor is aware of his/her own fears it may allow a fairer appreciation of the facts. An honest acknowledgement of the influence we have on patient decision-making should stop us from asking the patient to choose only when we cannot make up our own minds what to do and calling it patient autonomy.[101]

A patient-centred approach encourages us to understand the patient's value systems. What do they fear? What is important to them? Using sensitive communication we may make more appropriate decisions than by merely looking at survival statistics.[101]

In debating the benefit of a planned intervention, the possibility of an increase in survival or decreased long-term morbidity may be overridden by the certainty of valuable time wasted in hospital. The role of the doctor in palliative care is as a facilitator and teacher as much as diagnostician and decision maker.

Research offers another mechanism for coping with uncertainty. There is a need for qualitative research to explore the process and effects of medical, nursing and patient decision-making at the interface between curative and palliative care. Enhancing palliative care education at all levels of training is a necessary first step in changing doctors' behaviour. Hanson showed that educational interventions with physicians led to increased use of patient preferences, but sophisticated educational techniques were needed to motivate physicians to change their behaviour.[102]

This study has identified a variety of factors which contribute to the uncertainty felt by patients, relatives and professionals. The model derived from this study indicates the areas which need to be addressed if we are to help patients and their families to receive appropriate care.

---

**A MODEL FOR DECISION-MAKING
IN THE CARE OF PATIENTS WITH INCURABLE CANCER**

WORK IN A PARTNERSHIP    Patient...Family...Professionals

AGREE THE GOAL OF CARE    Curative to palliative

MAXIMISE QUALITY OF LIFE    Respect autonomy
Relief of symptoms
Maintain hope
Relieve suffering

---

**SHARE TREATMENT DECISIONS**

SEEK INFORMED CONSENT    Give honest information
Check that it is understood
No coercion
Allow time to think

EFFECTIVE DECISION-MAKING    Patient centred
Realistic
Acknowledge uncertainty

GOOD COMMUNICATION    Trust
Negotiation
Time
Continuity

## WHEN TO STOP PALLIATIVE CHEMOTHERAPY?

Quality of life

Effectiveness of palliation

Cost versus benefit

Acknowledge futility

Respect patient's choice

## PROVIDE APPROPRIATE CARE

Competence

Compassion

Commitment

# REFERENCES

1 Ashby M, Stofell B. Therapeutic ratio and defined phases: Proposal of an ethical framework for palliative care. *BMJ* 1991; 302: 1322-4.

2 Faithful S. The concept of cure in cancer care. *European Journal of Cancer Care* 1994; 3: 12-7.

3 Field D. Palliative medicine and the medicalisation of death. *European Journal of Cancer Care* 1994; 3: 58-62.

4 Illich I. *Limits to medicine. Medical nemesis: The expropriation of health.* London: Penguin 1990.

5 World Health Organisation. *Cancer pain relief and palliative care.* Report of a WHO expert committee (WHO Technical Report Series, 804) Geneva: World Health Organisation 1990.

6 George RJD, Jennings AL. Palliative Medicine. *Postgrad Med J* 1993; 69: 429-49.

7 Charlton R, Dovey S, Mizushima Y, Ford E. Attitudes to death and dying in the UK, New Zealand and Japan. *J Palliat Care* 1995; 11: 42-7.

8 Keen J, Packwood T. Case study evaluation. *BMJ* 1995; 311: 444-6.

9 Pope C, Mays N. Reaching the parts other methods cannot reach: An introduction to qualitative research methods in health and health services. *BMJ* 1995; 311: 42-5.

10 Silverman D. *Communication and medical practice*: London: Sage 1987.

11 Strong P. *The ceremonial order of the clinic*. London: Routledge 1989.

12 Mays N, Pope C. Observational methods in healthcare settings. *BMJ* 1995; 311: 182-4.

13 Mays N, Pope C. Rigour and qualitative research. *BMJ* 1995; 311: 109-12.

14 Reinharz S. *On becoming a social scientist: Transaction.* New Brunswick: 1984.

15 Bradley CP. Turning anecdotes into data: The critical incident technique. *Fam Pract* 1992; 9: 98-103.

16 Flanagan JC. The critical incident technique. *Psychology Bulletin* 1954; 51: 327-58.

17 Hurny C. Palliative care in high-tech medicine: Defining the point of no return. *Support Care Cancer* 1994; 2: 3-4.

18 Loescher LJ et al. Surviving adult cancers. Part 1: Physiological effects. *Ann Intern Med* 1989; 111: 411-32.

19 Shanfield S. On surviving cancer: Psychological considerations. *Comparative Psychiatry* 1980; 21: 128-34.

20 Quigley K. The adult cancer survivor: Psychosocial consequences of cure. *Semin Oncol Nurs* 1989; 5: 63-9.

21 Andersen B. Surviving cancer. *Cancer* 1994; 74: 1484-93.

22 Jeffrey D. *There is nothing more I can do*. Penzance: Patten Press, 1993.

23 Calman KC. Quality of life in cancer patients: An hypothesis. *J Med Ethics* 1984; 10: 124-7.

24 Twycross RG, Lichter I. The terminal phase. *Lancet* 1995: 345; 840-2.

25 Brody B. *Life and death decision-making*. New York: Oxford University Press, 1988.

26 Doyle D. Palliative medicine: A time for definition? *Palliat Med* 1993; 7: 253-5.

27  Roy DJ. Those days are long gone now. *J Palliat Care* 10: 2; 4-6.

28  Pennell M, Skevington S. Problems in conceptualising palliative care. In: *Teaching Palliative Care: Issues and implications*. Ed. MacLeod R, Jones C. Penzance: Patten Press 1994.

29  Coates A et al. Improving the quality of life during chemotherapy for advanced breast cancer. *N Engl J Med* 1987; 317: 1490-5.

30  Gelber RD, Goldhirsch, Cavalli F. Quality of life: Adjusted evaluation of adjuvant therapies for operable breast cancer. *Ann Intern Med* 1991; 114: 621-8.

31  Hoskins P, Makin W. *Oncology for Palliative Medicine*. Oxford University Press, 1998.

32  Slevin ML et al. Attitudes to chemotherapy: Comparing views of patients with cancer with those of doctors, nurses and general public. *BMJ* 300: 1458-60.

33  Meystre CJN et al. What investigations and procedures do patients in hospices want? Interview based survey of patients and their nurses. *BMJ* 1997; 315:1202-3.

34  Kearsley JH. Cytotoxic chemotherapy for common adult malignancies: 'The emperor's new clothes' revisited? *BMJ* 1986: 229; 871-6.

35  Gillon R. Medical ethics: Four principles plus attention to scope. *BMJ* 1994: 309; 184-8.

36  Cella DF. Measuring quality of life in palliative care. *Semin Oncol* 1995: 22 (suppl3); 73-81.

37  Sheldon F. *Psychosocial palliative care*. Cheltenham: Stanley Thornes, 1997.

38  Kaasa S et al. Prognostic factors for patients with inoperable non-small cell lung cancer. *Radiother Oncol* 1989: 15; 235-42.

39  Kukull WA et al. Symptom distress: Psychological variables and survival from lung cancer. *J Psychosocial Oncology* 1986: 4; 91-104.

40  Degner LF, Sloan JA. Symptom distress in newly diagnosed ambulatory cancer patients as a predictor in lung cancer. *J Pain Symptom Manage* 1995; 10: 423-31.

41  Regnard C. Judging prognosis in advanced disease. *CLIP: Current Learning in Palliative Care* June 1998.

42  Maltoni M et al. Prognostic factors in terminal cancer patients. *European Journal of Palliative Care* 1994; 1: 122-5.

43  Parkes CM. Accuracy of prediction of survival in later stages of cancer. *BMJ* 192; 2: 29-31.

44  Heyse-Moore LH. Can doctors accurately predict the life expectancy of patients with terminal cancer? *Palliat Med* 1987: 1; 165-6.

45  Reuben DB et al. Clinical symptoms and length of survival in patients with terminal cancer. *Arch Intern Med* 1988; 148: 1586-91.

46  Buchan JEF. Nurses' estimation of prognoses in the last days of life. *Int J Pall Nurs* 1995; 1: 12-6.

47  Forster LE, Lynn J. Predicting the life span for applicants to inpatient hospice. *Arch Intern Med* 1988; 148: 2540-3.

48  den Daas N. Estimating length of survival in end stage cancer: A review of the literature. *J Pain Symptom Manage* 1995; 10: 548-55.

49 Maltoni M et al. Clinical prediction of survival is more accurate than the Karnofsky performance status in estimating life span of terminally ill patients. *Eur J Cancer* 1994; 30A: 764-6.

50 Oxenham DR, Cornbleet MA. Accuracy of prediction of survival by different professional groups in a hospice. *Palliat Med* 1998; 12: 117-8.

51 Hardy JR et al. Prediction of survival in a hospital-based continuing care unit. *Eur J Cancer* 1994; 30A: 284-8.

52 Addington-Hall JM et al. Can the Spitzer Quality of Life Index help to reduce prognostic uncertainty in terminal care. *Br J Cancer* 1990; 62: 695-9.

53 Coates A et al. Prognostic value of quality of life score during chemotherapy for advanced breast cancer. *J Clin Oncol* 1992: 10; 1833-8.

54 Harvey KB et al. Nutritional assessment and patient outcome during oncological therapy. *Cancer* 1979; 43 (suppl): 2065-9.

55 Herrmann FR, et al. Serum albumen level on admission as a predictor of death, length of stay and readmission. *Arch Intern Med* 1992: 152; 125-30.

56 Phillips A et al. Association between serum albumen and mortality from cardiovascular disease, cancer and other causes. *Lancet* 1989; ii: 1434-6.

57 Rosenthal MA et al. Prediction of life expectancy in hospice patients: Identification of novel prognostic factors. *Palliat Med* 1993; 7: 199-204.

58 Cassileth BR et al. Psychosocial correlates of survival in advanced malignant disease. *N Eng J Med* 1985; 312: 1551-5.

59 Downie RS, Calman KC. *Healthy Respect*. London: Faber and Faber, 1987.

60 Fowlie M et al. Quality of life in advanced cancer: The benefits of asking the patient. *Palliat Med* 1989; 3: 55-9.

61 Gillon R. *Philosophical Medical Ethics*. Oxford: John Wiley, 1985.

62 Jeffrey D. Ethical issues in palliative care. In: *Handbook of Palliative Care*. Ed Faull C et al. Oxford: Blackwell, 1998.

63 Oxenham DR. Lessons from a symposium on palliative medicine. *Proc R Coll Physicians Edinb* 1995; 25: 569-73.

64 Townsend J et al. Terminal cancer care and patients' preference for place of death: A prospective study. *BMJ* 1990; 301: 415-7.

65 Cartwright A. Balance of care for the dying between hospitals and the community. *Br J Gen Pract* 1991; 41: 271-4.

66 Till JE et al. Is there a role for preference assessments in research on quality of life in oncology? *Qual Life Research* 1992; 1: 31-40.

67 Cherny NI et al. Suffering in the advanced cancer patient: A definition and taxonomy. *J Palliat Care* 1994; 10(2): 57-70.

68 Cassileth BR et al. Information and participation preferences among cancer patients. *Ann Intern Med* 1980; 92: 832-6.

69 Flemming K. The meaning of hope to palliative care cancer patients. *Int Journal Pall Nurs* 1997; 3: 14-8.

70 Dudgeon DJ et al. When does palliative care begin? A needs assessment of cancer patients with recurrent disease. *J Palliat Care* 1995; 11: 5-9.

71 Husebo S. Communication, autonomy and hope: How can we treat seriously ill patients with respect? In: Communication with the cancer patient: Information and truth. Ed Sunbane A et al. *Ann N Y Acad Sci* 1997.

72 Bursztajn HJ et al. *Medical choices, medical chances*. London: Routledge 1990.

73 Grundstein-Amado R. Ethical decision-making processes used by healthcare providers. *J of Adv Nurs* 1993; 18: 1701-9.

74 Macdonald N. Oncology and palliative care: The case for co-ordination. *Cancer Treat Rev* 1993; 19 (Suppl A): 29-41.

75 Donald AG. Palliative care in the community: Difficultics and dilemmas. *Proc R Coll Physicians Edinb* 1995; 25: 550-7.

76 Coulter A. Paternalism or partnership? *BMJ* 1999; 319: 719-20.

77 Howie JGR et al. Quality at general practice consultation: Cross sectional survey. *BMJ* 1999; 319: 738-43.

78 Hockley J. Rehabilitation in palliative care: Are we asking the impossible? *Palliat Med* 1993 (suppl 1), 9-15.

79 Moody HR. From informed consent to negotiated consent. *Gerontologist* 1988; 28: 64-70.

80 Towle A, Godolphin W. Framework for teaching and learning informed shared decision-making. *BMJ* 1999; 319: 766-71.

81 Edwards A et al. General practice registrar responses to the use of different risk communication tools in simulated consultations. *BMJ* 1999; 319: 749-52.

82 Charlton R et al. What do we mean by partnership in making decisions about treatment? *BMJ* 1999; 319: 780-2.

83 Field D. *Nursing the dying*. Tavistock: Routledge 1989.

84 Baum M et al. Ethics of clinical research: Lessons for the future. *BMJ* 1989; 299: 251-3.

85 Naylor C. Grey zones of clinical practice: Some limits to evidence-based medicine. *Lancet* 1995; 345: 840-2.

86 Schneiderman L et al. Medical futility: Its meaning and ethical implications. *Ann Intern Med* 1990; 112: 949-54.

87 Rubens RD et al. Appropriate chemotherapy for palliating advanced cancer. *BMJ* 1992; 304: 35-40.

88 Watson JV. What does response in cancer chemotherapy really mean? *BMJ* 1981; 283: 34-7.

89 Dyer C. Court confirms right to palliative treatment for mental distress. *BMJ* 1997; 315: 1178.

90 Meier DE et al. Improving palliative care. *Ann Intern Med* 1997; 127: 225-30.

91 Farsides CCS. Autonomy and its implications for palliative care: A northern European perspective. *Palliat Med* 1998; 12: 147-51.

92 Speck P. Power and autonomy in palliative care: A matter of balance. *Palliat Med* 1998; 12: 145-6.

93 Feynman R. Character of physical
laws. Cited in: Weschler L. *Mr
Wilson's cabinet of wonder*. New York:
Vintage Books 1996.

94 Dunlop R. Commentaries: When
palliative care fails to relieve
suffering. *J Palliat Care*. 1994; 10:
27-30.

95 Jeffrey D. Active euthanasia: Time
for a decision. *Br J Gen Pract* 1994;
44: 136-8.

96 Seale C. Social and ethical aspects of
euthanasia: A review. *Progress in
Palliative Care* 1997; 5: 141-6.

97 Jeffrey D Unrelieved suffering in
patients with advanced cancer: A
personal ethical perspective. *Proc R
Coll Physicians Edinb* 1998; 28: 535-
41.

98 Royal College of General
Practitioners and Cancer Relief
Macmillan Fund. *GP Facilitator
Project 1992-4*. 1995.

99 MacDonald N. The interface
between palliative medicine and
other hospital services. *Proc R Coll
Physicians Edinb* 1995; 25: 558-568.

100 Hanks GW. Difficult treatment
decisions in palliative care. *Eur J
Palliat Care* 1995; 1: 156.

101 Morphia. *Association of Palliative
Medicine Newsletter*. 1994; 15: 9.

102 Hanson C, Tulsky JA, Danis M. Can
clinical interventions change care at
the end of life? *Ann Intern Med* 1997;
126: 381-8.

103 Greer S. Cancer and the mind. *B J
Psychiatry* 1983; 143: 535-43.

104 Thorpe G. Enabling more dying
people to remain at home. *BMJ*
1993; 307: 915-8.

# *Ethical issues in palliative care*
## Reflections and considerations

Edited by **Patricia Webb**

This book brings together the knowledge and experience of a diverse team of professionals and raises questions surrounding the ethics of caring for people with progressive, life-limiting illness and their relatives.

Initial definitions and some theoretical discussion leads on to a practical text which will enable people from a variety of professions to discuss and debate issues further to their practice.

All contributors either work in palliative care, teach aspects of it, are conducting research in this area, or come into regular contact with people who have a progressive, life-limiting illness.

ISBN 1 898507 27 9

**£15.95**

Order by telephone: **0161 273 4156**

Please send me . . . . . copies of **ETHICAL ISSUES IN PALLIATIVE CARE** @ £15.95 each
UK postage free, for overseas postage please add 25% of total order value

☐ I enclose a cheque made payable to Hochland & Hochland Ltd

☐ Please debit my Visa/Mastercard/Switch/Delta

Card number

Issue number ............... Expiry date ........../.........
Signature .........................................................................................................................
Name .................................................................................................................................
Address .............................................................................................................................
.............................................................................................................................................
.............................................................................Postcode.....................................
Telephone ........................................................................................................................

Hochland & Hochland Ltd, University Precinct, Oxford Rd, Manchester M13 9QA

# Dying Well
## A guide to enabling a good death

### Julia Neuberger

What makes a good death? Rabbi Julia Neuberger gathers key viewpoints from the world's religions, cultures, philosophies and professions, to reach a new definition.

She encourages us all to consider our own expectations of death, and to express our hopes and fears so that our carers can help us achieve the death we want.

This book offers realistic yet empathetic advice to all those involved with caring for the dying, stressing the potential for death to be a tender, loving and spiritual experience. It also looks at the psychology of grief and tackles the fears and anger of those who are dying, their loved ones and their professional carers.

ISBN 1 898507 26 0

**£15.95**

Please send me . . . . . copies of **DYING WELL** @ £15.95 each
UK postage free, for overseas postage please add 25% of total order value

☐ I enclose a cheque made payable to Hochland & Hochland Ltd

☐ Please debit my Visa/Mastercard/Switch/Delta

Card number ☐☐☐☐☐☐☐☐☐☐☐☐☐☐☐☐☐☐☐

Issue number ............... Expiry date ........../..........
Signature ..............................................................................................................
Name ......................................................................................................................
Address ..................................................................................................................
...............................................................................................................................
...............................................................................................................................
.........................................................................Postcode.................................
Telephone ..............................................................................................................

Hochland & Hochland Ltd, University Precinct, Oxford Rd, Manchester M13 9QA

# Patient Information Series

The Royal Marsden's Patient Information booklets are designed to help the healthcare professional in patient education. Written by experienced clinical nurse specialists, these attractive and well-designed booklets give patients and their families factual and practical information about cancer, its diagnosis, treatment and care.

The booklets and leaflets can be purchased individually by patients or healthcare practitioners. Practitioners who wish to purchase copies in bulk for distribution to patients may claim a discount – see opposite. Practitioners can also obtain free copies of the Patient Information Series catalogue and price list from the address opposite.

All prices include postage and packing.

A pack of 25 booklets may be purchased for £50.00.
You may choose to order 25 of the same booklet or a mixture of booklets.

A pack of 50 leaflets may be purchased for £37.50.
You may choose to order 50 of the same leaflet or a mixture of leaflets.

You may also order an INTRODUCTORY PACK containing one copy of each title in the series for £60.00.

-- -- -- -- -- -- -- -- -- -- -- -- -- -- -- -- -- --

## ORDER FORM

| Number of item | Price per item | No of copies | Total £ |
|---|---|---|---|
| | | | |
| | | | |
| | | | |
| | | TOTAL £ | |

☐ I enclose a cheque payable to Hochland & Hochland Publications Ltd

☐ Please debit my Switch/Visa/Access card:

Card number: ☐☐☐☐☐☐☐☐☐☐☐☐☐☐☐☐☐☐

Expiry date: ........................    Issue number (Switch only): ....................

Name:.....................................................................................

Address:..................................................................................

.............................................................................................

Telephone:...............................................................................

*Send your order to:*

Hochland & Hochland Publications Ltd
The University Precinct, Oxford Road, Manchester M13 9QA

*Or contact us by telephone, fax or email to place a credit card order.*

Hochland & Hochland Publications Ltd
Telephone 0161 273 4156
Fax 0161 273 4340
Email sales@hochland.demon.co.uk